Exhausted & Drained?

It's **NOT** Just in Your Brain.

Identify and Heal from Adrenal Stress and Fatigue to Regain Your Energy

Kerry Sauser ARNP, ND, PhD

First published by Dog Ear Publishing
4010 W. 86th Street, Ste H
Indianapolis, IN 46268
www.dogearpublishing.net

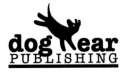

ISBN: 978-1-4575-1046-5

This book is printed on acid-free paper.

Printed in the United States of America

INTRODUCTION

Although exact numbers are unavailable, it is estimated that more than 30 million individuals may be suffering from adrenal stress and fatigue. Could this be you? Do you suffer from fatigue unrelieved by rest, depression, and mental fog, lack of interest in sex, insomnia, weight gain, or fibromyalgia? While many of these symptoms may be attributed to an unhealthy lifestyle, chronic stress, and/or poor nutrition, this may also indicate adrenal stress or fatigue. Part I of this book answers basic questions for the informed patient who seeks healing from adrenal stress and fatigue.

- ❖ What actually is this condition?
- ❖ How do I know I have it?
- ❖ Why has my doctor not told me?
- ❖ What should I do about it?
- ❖ Where should I go for help?
- ❖ How do I develop a self-care plan?
- ❖ How do I locate a healthcare provider for assistance?
- ❖ What should I expect in a recovery program?
- ❖ How can I prevent this condition?

Part II of this book is written for health care providers to share with their patients. It offers insights regarding diagnosis and therapy for patients with adrenal stress and fatigue, and is based on this author's PhD (nutrition) dissertation as well as my 43 years of clinical experience in Western and integrative health care. The final chapter of this book includes a summary of the research conducted while completing the dissertation. This research was based on a sampling of individuals—mostly from the Midwest—who were evaluated with medical and dietary histories. In addition, all individuals were asked to complete a symptom survey and undergo appropriate testing.

A literature review supporting the information included is provided. The resulting dissertation analysis indicates two hypotheses. The first states that individuals making unhealthy nutritional choices (especially those with carbohydrate cravings) have above average problems with adrenal stress and fatigue when compared to their counterparts. The second indicates that good nutritional guidelines, reduced stress and appropriate lifestyle changes, along with the support of nutritional supplements and herbs, can improve the subject's health.

❖ Disclaimer: The information in this book is designed for education only. It contains information on Standard Process, MediHerb and NSA, LLC products but is not the expressed opinion of Standard Process, MediHerb or NSA. Standard Process is the exclusive distributor of MediHerb in the United States. MediHerb and Standard Process are registered trademarks of MediHerb Pty., Ltd. and Standard Process, Inc., respectively. MediHerb and Standard Process expressly disclaim any responsibility for and make no representation or warranties regarding any statement, information, materials or content found on or included in this publication. Herbal products are plant-based and designed to support the body— not to treat any disease. The information enclosed is not designed as a substitute for medical advice. Please see a qualified healthcare provider for further assistance.

DEDICATION AND ACKNOWLEDGEMENTS

To my husband, Robert, whose unconditional love and support have not only made this book possible, but have also enabled me to develop the Complementary Care Center and my practice, the Natural Health Center. I also thank the physicians at Diagnos-Techs, Inc for providing me a grant for the Adrenal Stress Index Tests and also thank Marilyn and Susan for their assistance and friendship throughout the years. Most of all, I thank God for leading me down this path to help others, for opening doors and bringing the right people into my life at just the right time. Lastly, I would like to thank all my patients who have taught me so much.

TABLE OF CONTENTS

LIST OF ABBREVIATIONS

CAD   Coronary Artery Disease

CRH   Corticotrophin releasing hormone

CVD   Cardiovascular Disease

DHEA   Dehydroepiandrosterone

GERD   Gastro Esophageal Reflux Disease

HPA axis   Hypothalamus-pituitary-adrenal axis

IBS   Irritable Bowel Syndrome

IRB   Institutional Review Board

LDL   Low Density Lipoprotein

LH   Luteinizing Hormone

PS   Phosophatidylserine

PMG   Protomorphogen

PMS   Pre Menstrual Syndrome

SAD   Standard American Diet

SIgA   Secretory IgA

PART ONE:

TO THE INFORMED PATIENT

CHAPTER 1

What is Adrenal Stress and Fatigue?

CURRENT RESEARCH INDICATES that millions of individuals are suffering from stress-related illnesses. These illnesses may include hypertension, cardiovascular disease, cancer, and headaches, as well as gastrointestinal problems, such as ulcers and gastro esophageal reflux disease (GERD), depression, chronic fatigue, and fibromyalgia which are more prevalent in today's world. Adrenal stress/fatigue is frequently the underlying cause of all these conditions.

Western medicine is very good at diagnosis and sick care, however, it appears inadequate in properly evaluating or recommending natural approaches for preventing illness, or for assisting individuals in their healing process. While numerous natural health and functional medicine practitioners are studying adrenal stress/fatigue, many Western medicine practitioners fail to recognize the existence of these conditions. Dr. James Wilson (2001) notes that, "despite the development of the first effective treatment [of adrenal fatigue] in the 1930s, most "conventional" physicians are unaware that the problem exists!" (p.xi)

The Mayo Clinic reinforces this with an official stance stating, "Adrenal fatigue is a label applied to a collection of nonspecific symptoms, such as body aches, fatigue, nervousness, sleep disturbances, and digestive problems. Although this term often shows up in popular health books and alternative medicine websites, it isn't an accepted medical diagnosis" (Mayo Clinic Staff, 2007). The Mayo Clinic's view on adrenal fatigue was unchanged when the site was visited in 2011.

Based on research and my clinical experience it is my belief that adrenal stress and fatigue exists as a specific medical condition. It is an underlying cause of many illnesses, even though it is currently not recognized as an official health issue by Western medicine. In fact, over the last ten years, my practice has seen an increasingly large number of individuals whose underlying problems are adrenal stress and fatigue. High adrenal fatigue features low cortisol and severe hormone depletions. To support the theory that Western medicine does not seem to recognize subclinical adrenal issues, Baker (2005) states that:

> standard medical thinking regarding adrenal glands is like that of other organ systems in the body; that is, they are either considered to be in satisfactory working order, or they are in failure. Rarely is the diagnosis made of hypo function in any organ system, without the presence of notable pathologic tissue changes and function. (p. 259)

Nippoldt (2009), Mayo Clinic endocrinologist, further states the Western view on adrenal fatigue:

> Proponents of the adrenal fatigue diagnosis claim this is a mild form of adrenal insufficiency caused by chronic stress. The unproven theory behind adrenal fatigue is that your adrenal glands are unable to keep pace with demands of perpetual flight-or- fight arousal. As a result, they can't produce quite enough of the hormones you need to feel good.

Consequently, Western medicine may only diagnose end-stage adrenal diseases such as Cushing's disease and Addison's disease. In contrast to this view, professionals following functional/natural health protocols can often isolate subclinical problems earlier giving clients additional alternatives to those offered by many Western practitioners. With this information in mind, I have chosen to complete a literature review regarding adrenal stress and fatigue in both Western medicine and functional/natural health protocols.

Background and History

The first step in evaluating and providing therapy for a condition is to understand the problem. Adrenal fatigue, first noted in medical texts in the 1800s, has been largely ignored by Western medicine (Wilson, 2001). However, as early as 1926, Dr. Hans Selye began to study the stress response. Selye speculated that stress was the basis of most disease and labeled good stress "eustress" and bad or negative stress "distress" (National Center for Complementary and Alternative Medicine, 2005). According to the Canadian Institute of Stress, stress disability rates have doubled from 1995 to 2004 with the top stressor being the juggling of work and family life of two working parents (Selye, 2008). The number of prescriptions for antidepressants and minor tranquilizers now equals that of drugs for hypertension and cardiovascular disease (CVD). This is evident on countless television ads.

Incidence of Adrenal Fatigue

Although it is impossible to tell the full incidence of adrenal stress and fatigue, from this author's research and experience, it is likely that millions of individuals may suffer from the underlying adrenal burnout and are sick and tired of being sick and tired. These individuals may have problems with hypoglycemia (low blood sugar), fatigue unrelieved by rest, depression, irritability, anxiety, digestive problems, cardiovascular disease (CVD), obesity, and hypothyroidism. Genetics may also play a part in adrenal stress and fatigue. According to Wilson (2001), adrenals may be weak from birth if the mother has adrenal fatigue. Those children are therefore less able to cope with stress in their own lives. In addition, Entring, Kumsta, Hellhammer, Wadhwa, and Wust (2009) completed a study that "provides first evidence in humans of an association between prenatal psychosocial stress exposure and subsequent alterations in the regulation of the HPA axis" (hypothalamus-pituitary-adrenal) (p.292).

Anatomy and Physiology of Adrenal Stress and Fatigue

Adrenal stress and fatigue involves the adrenal glands, which are two walnut- sized endocrine glands that sit atop each kidney (Norman Endocrine Surgery Clinic, 2002b). These orange-colored glands consist of the cortex (outer layer) and the medulla (center). The adrenal medulla produces epinephrine (adrenalin) and norepinephrine (noradrenalin). Epinephrine increases heart rate, blood flow to the muscles and brain, and relaxation of smooth muscles, as well as assisting with the conversion of glycogen in the liver. Norepinephrine causes vasoconstriction of blood vessels, which in turn can raise blood pressure but has little effect on cardiac output and muscle function. These two hormones—-epinephrine and norepinephrin—- are neurotransmitters that activate the fight- or-flight response (Lang, 2004).

Traditional Chinese Medicine teaches that the kidney/adrenal channels are where life force begins. Therefore, the adrenals are important for our body's response to emotions of anger, fear, excitement and surprise (Gorman, 2004). In addition, the adrenal glands are important in the blood for maintaining normal blood sugar. Since high cortisol increases blood sugar, it can lead to higher insulin levels. Increased insulin levels cause free radicals which can damage the brain's hippocampus (Pawlak, 2007). Cortisol also has powerful anti-inflammatory qualities, affects the immune system, and causes constriction of mid-sized arteries.

The adrenal cortex produces many hormones including dehydroepiandrosterone (DHEA), pregnenolone, progesterone, estrogen, testosterone, cortisol, and aldosterone. DHEA is an androgen, or male hormone, with anabolic activity that builds tissues activity. DHEA is a precursor to testosterone and estrogen. It serves five purposes: reversing immune suppression caused by excess cortisol, and stimulating bone remodeling to prevent osteoporosis, lowers total cholesterol and low-density lipoprotein (LDL) levels, and increases muscle mass while decreasing body fat. Lastly, cortisol synthesized from cholesterol is stimulated by the pituitary adrenocorticotropic hormone (ACTH) which in turn is regulated by corticotrophin releasing factor (CRF). The level of cortisol affects appetite, amount of body fat, muscle mass, bone density, anxiety, depression, mood swings, libido, immune system, and memory. (See chart on adrenal hormone pathway.)

CHAPTER 2

Am I at Risk?

IN ORDER TO identify and provide therapy for adrenal stress and fatigue, knowledge of what can affect the adrenal glands is important. These influences include:

- ❖ Emotions such as anger, fear, worry, and guilt
- ❖ Overwork with physical or emotional strain
- ❖ Unwanted unemployment
- ❖ Financial concerns
- ❖ Excessive or lack of exercise
- ❖ Change in health, surgery, trauma, illness, or injury
- ❖ Unhealthy diet including white sugar, white flour, and junk foods
- ❖ Excessive use of caffeinated beverages or other stimulants
- ❖ Exposure to toxins or other chemicals
- ❖ Lack of sleep or irregular sleep patterns
- ❖ Poor digestion
- ❖ Hypoglycemia
- ❖ Excessive use of prescription or non-prescription drugs
- ❖ Unhappy marriage or other relationship
- ❖ Death of a loved one (Wilson, 2001)

Lifestyle and events leading up to adrenal stress/fatigue:

- All work, no play
- Shift work causing irregular sleeping patterns
- Single parent with two or more children and poor support system
- Stressful work environment
- Starting a new business
- Frequent crisis at home or work
- Major surgery
- Prolonged or repeated illnesses (which can cause hypothalamic suppression)
- Moving to new location without support of family or friends (Wilson, 2001).

Typical Signs and Symptoms of Adrenal Stress and Fatigue

There are many symptoms of adrenal fatigue, so it is impossible to estimate the percentage of Americans who have adrenal fatigue. A common client complaint is, "I am so tired no matter how much rest I get. My doctor thinks I'm depressed, but I am just tired." Other complaints are often of weight gain and lack of interest in sex. The most frequent complaints of an individual with adrenal fatigue are:

- Fatigue not relieved by rest
- Craving of sweets for quick energy
- Fatigue/cravings after meals
- Decreased ability to handle stress
- Reduced or diminished sex drive
- Slow starter in the morning
- Lightheaded when rising from a sitting or lying down position
- Brain fog
- Difficulty sleeping
- Feeling better briefly after a meal or snack
- Needing stimulants (coffee, soda, tea) in the morning
- Gastrointestinal distress (stomach burning and ulcers)

❖ Leaky gut
❖ Pre-menstrual Syndrome (PMS)
❖ Osteoporosis
❖ Yeast infections
❖ Tendency to stay up late until one gets his second wind
❖ High blood pressure (adrenal stress)
❖ Low blood pressure (adrenal fatigue)
❖ Inability to cope with life stressors
❖ Tendency to gain weight and difficulty losing it
❖ Poor immune system
❖ Mild depression
❖ Fears, phobias, and anxiety (Wilson, J., 2001)

While individuals having symptoms of adrenal stress and fatigue in manageable situations is natural, those remaining in prolonged stress response with high cortisol levels may develop problems with poor control of the hypothalamus, pituitary, adrenal (HPA) axis. If this happens, the ability to slow down and relax is impaired. Repairing the HPA axis is necessary for healing. In addition, damage to the hippocampus can result from prolonged stress leading to memory and mood problems and may lead to dementia.

This can then cause a decrease in both male and female hormones leading to deficiencies and estrogen dominance (Lang, 2007). Elevated cortisol can decrease thyroid hormone production, which, in turn, slows metabolism. Sugar cravings and insulin resistance can follow causing cortisol to surge. This results in increasing fatigue.

High cortisol levels can also cause other conditions such as decreased ability to cope with stress and difficulty sleeping. Elevated evening cortisol levels can cause decreased SIgA (immune system of the GI tract), which causes a decrease in immune system function. This damage to the GI (gastrointestinal) system can then cause conditions such as stomach burning, leaky gut, dysbiosis (deficiency of good bacteria and overgrowth of harmful bacteria in the gut), ulcers, irritable bowel syndrome, and yeast or parasite infections. Noting all the commercials advertising drugs to treat GI problems further points toward current increases in adrenal stress/fatigue. Elevated cortisol can cause two other health problems. First, elevated cortisol pulls calcium and magnesium from bones and may lead to osteoporosis. Secondly, when cortisol levels remain high, the liver has difficulty metabolizing and excreting hormones.

In addition to the above, high cortisol levels may cause a decrease in luteinizing hormone (LH) production resulting in progesterone deficiency and premenstrual syndrome (PMS) or estrogen dominance in women. In men, suppression of LH can lead to declining testosterone and loss of androgen dominance. Ahrens, Deuschie, Krumm, van der Pompe, den Boer, and Lederbogen (2008) found that women with recurrent major depression disorder had evidence of HPA axis hyperactivity in both baseline state and when stressed.

In summary, acute adrenal stress features are high stress, elevated cortisol, sleep disturbances, and a suppressed immune system. Mild adrenal fatigue features irregular cortisol rhythm along with hormone irregularities. High adrenal fatigue features low cortisol and severe hormone depletions. The same symptoms may appear in individuals having low cortisol levels and those having high cortisol levels. These symptoms include GI problems, difficulty handling stress, and an impaired immune system. Therefore, complete, extensive evaluations are required for accurate assessment and successful therapy of individuals. Additionally, individuals may also have a problem with low blood sugar, difficulty staying asleep, dysfunction of the HPA axis, and inflammation (Pawlak, 2007; Eck, 1993).

CHAPTER 3

The Long Road to Exhaustion

STRESS (THE "FIGHT or flight" response) involves several steps. First, the sympathetic nervous system causes a release of epinephrine by the adrenal medulla. This, in turn, stimulates the hypothalamus-pituitary-adrenal (HPA) axis to release ACTH, which then stimulates the adrenal cortex to increase cortisol. Humans are designed for this short-term, well-managed stress, however, long-term or chronic stress damages the body in various ways.

As commonly stated in research regarding stress, Selye, known as the father of stress research, described the three stages of stress called the General Adaptation Syndrome. In Stage 1 or alarm stage, the body prepares for the threat called "fight or flight." During this stage the ACTH, cortisol, and DHEA are elevated, but they remain in balance. If the stress continues, Stage 2 begins. This is the resistance phase in the body that develops resistance to stress since the body cannot stay in "fight or flight." Individuals in the resistance phase usually develop adrenal insufficiency, which decreases DHEA and total cortisol. At this time, the cortisol to DHEA ratio is elevated. In Stage 3, stress has now become chronic and the body becomes exhausted. In this stage both cortisol and DHEA are low (Ilyia p.9).

Chronic stress, caused by real or imagined threats, ages the brain (especially the hippocampus) leading to premature aging of the brain and a number of diseases (Pawlak, 2007; Leventhal, 1998). The hippocampus is an area in the limbic system that records and stores long-term memory, which is important to memory and learning. According to Pawlak, most stress is psychological as is caused by thinking about threats, rather than the actual physical threats themselves. Repeatedly initiating the stress response or staying in a prolonged stress response causes bodily damage. Chronic stress causes increased heart rate, blood pressure, and elevated blood sugar and insulin. These can lead to coronary artery disease, high blood pressure, increased abdominal obesity, increased insulin resistance, diabetes and decreased immune response (Pawlak, 2007).

While many current Western medicine physicians are unskilled in diagnosing adrenal stress and fatigue as an underlying cause of many patients' complaints they are skilled at diagnosing the two end stages of adrenal diseases (Addison's disease and Cushing's disease). Addison's disease is a hormone deficiency of adrenal cortex, in which cortisol and sodium levels are low. Autoimmune diseases, infections, hemorrhages, tumors, or anticoagulants may cause this deficiency. Risk factors related to Addison's disease may include diabetes, diseases of the pituitary and parathyroid, Grave's disease, inflammation of the thyroid, chronic yeast infection, pernicious anemia, or testicular dysfunction. Tests to rule out these conditions may include abdominal x-ray, CT scan, and various lab tests. If these tests are positive for Addison's disease, the condition is treated with corticosteroids for the rest of the individual's life (U.S. National Library of Medicine, National Institutes of Health, 2004).

The second end-stage adrenal disease—Cushing's disease—is also a disease of the adrenal cortex. This condition results in excessive cortical production. This may result in abdominal obesity, high blood pressure, excessive hair growth, osteoporosis, and menstrual irregularity. A CT scan or a MRI may help determine the diagnosis of Cushing's disease but additional testing may be needed. Therapy for Cushing's disease depends on the cause. In the case of tumors, surgery is one option. Another option is drug therapy which may have limited effectiveness.

CHAPTER 4

My Doctor Says It's All in My Head!

TODAY THE AVERAGE patient is not well informed on lifestyle changes needed to reverse health problems after they appear, or better yet, prevent them from occurring. Western medicine is a practice of sick care and it offers little or nothing for maintaining health because its practitioners are mostly educated in controlling rather than addressing underlying causes of disease and discomfort. Drug deficiencies or surgical procedures are not the cause of diseases and illnesses. While there is a time and place for drugs and surgery, doing so often masks symptoms and sets the stage for more serious problems down the line. In addition, another drug may be added to control the side effects of a previously prescribed drug. In 1900 30% of our population suffered from chronic degenerative disease, while today 70% of the United States population suffers from one or more chronic diseases. This continues to increase as the population ages in spite of popular drug and surgery protocols.

Typically Western medicine protocols largely ignore the first step in helping the client heal, which is to evaluate the client's nutritional status. This practice makes sense to Western medicine because this philosophy often places the function of organs in either of two categories––they are working satisfactorily or they are failing. An organ working in a suboptimal state is often not considered (Barker, 2005). This observation is reinforced by the findings from an internet search for nutritional education courses offered in ten medical schools located in different regions of the country from the Association of American

Medical Colleges' *Tomorrows Doctors* [2006]). This search shows only two schools offering nutritional courses. Albany Medical College located in Albany, New York, has an impressive nutritional program that includes two 30-week courses and one 9-week course in nutrition in their curriculum. The Lucille A. Craver College of Medicine at the University of Iowa offered 16 hours or a one week course in case-based lectures on nutrition. The remaining eight medical schools from various areas of the United States had no nutrition programs in their curriculums. The aforementioned website was again visited in January 2010 looking at the graduation year of 2012. Albany Medical College again listed the same nutrition courses, while the Lucille A. Craver College of Medicine at the University of Iowa no longer listed their nutrition courses. Bayer College of Medicine now lists a nutrition course but does not mention the number of hours. The University of Missouri Columbia added nutrition with a month block included as Pathophysiology of Diseases: Nutrition, Cardiovascular, Respiratory, and Blood, the University of California listed a three-month course called "Metabolism and Nutrition". The other schools previously researched have no new nutritional courses listed.

On the other hand, Functional medicine attempts to prevent disease and strives to reverse and halt an existing disease. If the disease cannot be reversed, then the goal is to improve quality of life with the disease. Functional medicine sees symptoms as a friend or a signal to get our attention. If given the right tools the body can bring about healing. Several recognized researchers attest to this theory. In the early 1900s Dr. Royal Lee, DDS (born in 1885) was already a researcher, inventor, scientist, and a pioneer in the study of nutrition. He felt the underlying cause of many health problems was poor nutrition. Dr. Lee spent his own money researching and discovering the causes of good health, rather than the cause of disease. He believed the whole was greater than the sum of its parts, and that the whole was a functioning mechanism that had characteristics well beyond chemical components. As Dr Lee stated, "What part of a watch keeps time? No part does, but it only works well in combination with the other parts."

Dr. Lee developed many nutritional supplements to help assist the body in the healing process and is the founder of Standard Process (a whole food supplement company located in Palmyra, Wisconsin). Lee stated, "Nature produces plant complexes with known and unknown components that function synergistically, which in the animal produce the vitamin effect. Just as the chemist cannot create, neither can he create a complex vitamin: the life element in foods and nutrition. This is a mystery the chemist has never solved and probably never will, and the synthetic vitamins he creates on the basis of chemical formulae bear as much resemblance to the real thing as a robot does to a living man, lacking an elusive quality that chemistry cannot supply."

Lee developed many products, but two were especially formulated for healing of the adrenal glands. These products were Drenamin® and Drenatrophin PMG®. Drenamin® contains Cataplex ®C (whole food vitamin C), Cataplex® G (niacin riboflavin, ascorbic acid) and Drenatrophin PMG® (bovine adrenal PMG). In his writings Lee related nutritional deficiency to a physical breakdown. His information went mostly unnoticed by Western medicine in fact, the FDA persecuted him for his efforts. At that time, the FDA labeled Dr. Lee a racketeer because he promoted whole food nutrition from natural food with all its vitamins, minerals, and enzymes intact (Farr, 2001). Dr. Lee stated, "Innovators are rarely received with joy, and established authorities launch into condemnation of newer truths, for…at every crossroads to the future there are a thousand self-appointed guardians of the past."

In 1997-1999, Wetzel, Eisenberg and Kaptchukl conducted a study on CAM (complementary and alternative medicine) in United States medical schools. This group contacted 125 medical schools with 117 replying. Of those schools, 64 percent offered elective courses in complementary or alternative medicine or had some topics in required courses. Chiropractic, acupuncture, homeopathy, herbs, and mind body techniques were some of the topics covered, but there was no mention of any nutrition classes. Cohen, Sandler, Hrbek, Davis, and Eisenberg (2005) studied polices regarding complementary and alternative therapies in 39 academic health centers. They found only 23 offered some CAM services while only 10% had written policies regarding use of dietary supplements. According to Trindle, Davis, Russell, Phillips and Eisenberg (2005) the use of CAM remained the same between 1997 and 2002. Greater than 1 in 3 representing about 72 million adults use some form of CAM (Complementary/Alternative Medicine). The public has heard of many systems of medicine. Please see "Definition of Terms" at the end of this book for further information on these systems.

CHAPTER 5

Why It's NOT Your Imagination!

IN THIS CHAPTER, we will define adrenal stress and fatigue and its causes, and compare beliefs of Western medicine and Functional medicine regarding this condition and its effect on other body systems. In the following chapter, we will discuss the tools available to identify this condition.

Two major factors may cause or contribute to adrenal stress and fatigue and may occur at the same time. One of these factors is lifestyle. Examples of life style issues are university student, mother with multiple children, single parent, unhappy marriage, unhappy or stressful working environment, alcohol or drug abuser, alternating shift work, and all work and no play. A second factor is life events such as unrelieved pressure or frequent crisis at work or home, severe emotional trauma, death of a close friend or family member, major surgery, prolonged illness, serious burns, head trauma, loss of stable job, and sudden change of financial status. Repeated chemical exposure and other factors, which include allergies, smoking, poor eating habits, lack of or too much exercise, excessive caffeine intake, and fear can also contribute to this condition (Wilson, 2001, p.12-18)

Stress

The following reviews illustrate how chronic stress can affect the subject's health. Gorman's (2004) article on fight or flight explains how modern life has changed from a simpler way of life to "a hot-wired, high stakes game of mental challenge and response that is played at break-neck speeds and has become daily life in the United States and is mak-ing us sick." (p.1) When the "flight or fight" response occurs, the body prepares for danger by secreting epinephrine from the adrenal medulla, which then stimulates the HPA (hypothalamus-pituitary-adrenals) axis to release ACTH causing the adrenal cortex to release cortisol. When this becomes a chronic condition, "researchers found that all-cause mor-tality was 63% higher in caregivers who were under constant stress" (Kiecolt-Glaser, 2003). In addition, Roy-Byrne comments (regarding Bierhaus (2003) study of 19 subjects who preformed stressful tasks before an audience) that chronic stress affects various diseases such as "cardiovascular illness and immune dysfunction" (as cited in Bierhaus, 2003, p.1920).

In addition, Cohen (1991) also completed a study showing "psy-chological stress was significantly correlated with the development of cold symptoms," and that the greater the stress the more likely an infec-tion developed (p.606). Roy-Byrne comments regarding a study com-pleted by Carpenter (2004) on depressed patients showed they "generally experience more exposures to stress than nondepressed indi-viduals." (p.777). Another study showed that those with higher stress could die 9 to 17 years sooner than others (Epel, 2004). Environmen-tal stressors such as weather, noise, pollution, and radiation from cell phones, computers, electrical equipment, power lines, and air travel are additional stressors.

Lifestyle

We have determined stress is one of the causes of adrenal stress and fatigue. When we discuss stress and the adrenals, we are not just talking about what is happening today but what has happened over the years: "How long has it been since you felt well?" "Have you been exhausted for years with all you are doing?" Let us start with today's children. How many activities are they involved in? Are they allowed time to play? Are they involved in multiple sports activities, dance classes, or clubs such as scouts? Are there activities every evening to attend? Think about the average teen—parents want them to do well in school, have a part-time job and be involved in sports or other club activities! Often these teens are operating on a less-than- optimal diet, which further stresses the individual. Sadly, these lifestyles are increasingly producing teens who become very overwhelmed, exhausted young adults.

When a typical young adult leaves home, he or she may look for a job, struggle to balance finances, and often work in a demanding job while attending a graduate program. Many young adults marry and start families in addition to the above-mentioned activities thus increasing responsibilities and more stress.

Older persons may experience stress in living frugally, trying to balance budgets, or cope with additional health concerns. Losing a lifelong mate can also increase stress for the elderly.

The following study shows lifestyles effect on stress. It was conducted in 1999 and "compared health statistics and factors influencing the health of populations that had previously lived under different political systems." (Hillen, 1999) A sample of 4,430 Berlin residents over 18 were asked to rate their health. "Residents of East Berlin rated their health more frequently more unsatisfactory than residents of West Berlin." The authors looked at life events, social support, education, and health promoting lifestyle (Hillen, 1999). Another study conducted in 1996, done on nurses working both days and night shifts, found that the "pituitary-adrenal responses to corticotrophin releasing hormone (CRH) are markedly disrupted after only 5 days of nighttime work" (Leese, 1996). Unfortunately, compared to 1996, nurses are now required to work longer shifts and care for more critically ill patients because there are fewer staff members to do the same amount of work. As a whole, individuals who work in health care or in the ministry are deeply caring people. Because they give so much to others, they often develop adrenal stress or burn out.

Nutrition and the Adrenal Glands

To work effectively and efficiently adrenals need specific nutrients best found in food or whole food supplements. Vitamin B5, a part of the CoA enzyme, is used by the adrenal cortex as part of the production of glucocorticoids and other adrenal hormones. Vegetables, egg yolks, brewer's yeast, fish, and chicken all contain Vitamin B5. Another important vitamin needed by the adrenals is Vitamin C found in fruits and vegetables. On average, the adrenals store up to 30 mg of Vitamin C. (This emphasizes the importance of this vitamin to the adrenals). Since Vitamin C is water-soluble it needs to be consumed daily (Barker, 2005). The average American's daily intake of fruits, vegetables, and fast foods (as shown below) is proof of why diet plays a major part in adrenal stress/fatigue.

According to the CDC (2007), a diet high in fruits can decrease the risk for chronic disease. Data from 26 states showed greater than 30% of adults ate two or more servings of fruits a day (range from 19.2% to 37.8%) while ten states reported 30% of adults ate vegetables three or more times per day (range 20.9% to 39%). Diets lacking in fruits and vegetables cause many nutritional disorders including a weakened immune system, retardation, cancer, and cardiovascular disease. Many guidelines recommend five or more servings of fruits and vegetables daily, but nine or ten daily servings are preferred. (Food and Drug Organization of the United Nations, 2003).Those involved in intense sports may require up to 20 servings of fruits and vegetables daily. The CDC (2003) also looked at all fifty states and territories rating them on the number of adults who consumed five or more fruits and vegetables daily. The U.S. Virgin Islands rated 33.9% and Puerto Rico was rated the lowest at 23.1%.

Since 1970, the intake of fast foods has increased 300% with the largest increase in the 10 to 39 age groups. The intake of breads, cereals, fruits and vegetables were lower in those teens who ate fast food (Sullivan, 2003). Fast foods for the most part, contain no milk, fruit, or important key nutrients, yet they typically provide one-third of all calories consumed.

These examples illustrate how recent dietary trends have led to food choices with lower nutrient density. Because of our soils changing content, conventionally grown foods today have lower nutrient density than in the past, and now contain as much as one-forth tone-half the trace minerals of organically grown foods. Modern food processing damages or removes many nutrients. One example is white bread. Whole grain wheat arrives at the factory where it is stripped of most of its nutrients by removing the bran and germ, then the flour is bleached to make it whiter. At this point, a few vitamins are added back to the flour so it can be labeled "enriched". When food containing highly processed white flour is eaten, it robs nutrients from the body just to process it. In addition, many foods are genetically modified, which may contribute to digestion and absorption difficulties. The more foods are processed, the more their natural enzymes are destroyed. Common deficiencies in the American Standard Diet (SAD) consumed today are iron, vitamin C, Vitamin E, Vitamin D, zinc, and Omega 3 essentially fatty acids. Recommended Daily Allowances (RDAs) only recommend the amounts of nutrients needed to prevent deficiencies, not optimal health.

Obesity is one of the results of eating a SAD diet and the nutritional deficiencies it causes. The Vital Signs report, recently released by the Centers for Disease Control (CDC), shows about 2.4 million more adults were obese in 2009 than in 2007. This report was based on a telephone survey of 400,000 people, and the numbers were frightening! In fact, more than 72 million U.S. adults—or 26.7 percent—are now obese. In nine states, including those in the South and Midwest, (the "Stroke Belt") more than 30% of adults were obese. Medical care costs associated with obesity now total about $147 billion. Dr. Thomas Frieden, director of the CDC states, "If we don't change, more people will get sick and die from obesity-related conditions such as heart disease, stroke, type 2 diabetes and certain types of cancer, which are some of the leading causes of death."

CHAPTER 6

How Do I Know For Sure That I Have Adrenal Stress or Fatigue?

Client History

WHETHER A HEALTH care provider works in Western medicine, in a naturopathic role, or in functional medicine, a primary way or first tool for evaluating clients is by taking and recording the clients' histories as well as their chief complaints. Tattersall (1999) states that the existence of a milder form of Addison's disease is "characterized by weakness, lethargy, low blood pressure, and gastric irritability." These are also common characteristics of adrenal stress and fatigue (p 450). There are numerous books and websites devoted to adrenal stress and fatigue in which these symptoms are used for determining the possible existence of adrenal stress and fatigue such as Wilson's book, *Adrenal Fatigue,* and Hart's book, *Adrenaline and Stress,* and websites such as *Women to Women* and *Dr. Lam.* An article printed in the *Townsend Letter* entitled "The Naturopathic Approach to Adrenal Dysfunction," echoes these same sentiments. Several additional tests may also be used to evaluate the patient's condition.

When patients complain of fatigue, Western medicine providers will often evaluate for conditions such as sleep apnea, diabetes, hypothyroidism, or anemia. Screening for these conditions includes patient history and serum blood screens such as complete blood count, blood sugar, and free T3, T4, thyroid-stimulating hormone (TSH), and thyroid antibodies. In addition, if sleep apnea is a consideration, a sleep study may be completed. Many times these tests are within normal limits, even though adrenal stress/fatigue indications are not, and clients are told that nothing is wrong, or they are placed on antidepressants and their underlying conditions are seldom, if ever addressed.

Systems Survey

Besides patient history, many providers gain additional information by asking their clients to complete a systems survey form. The client rates various symptoms according to frequency of occurrence. The number one is circled if the symptom occurs once or twice a month or is mild, the number two is circled for symptoms that occur weekly or are moderate and the number three is circled for a symptom which occurs daily or is severe. The survey is divided into eight groups with one section being used for the male or female systems. An area is also provided for the client to write his or her five main physical complaints. The most common complaint noted in these surveys at my practice is fatigue, followed by brain fog and lack of interest in sex.

Saliva Testing

The next tool, in addition to the client history and systems survey is saliva testing. All humans are subject to stress, especially in todays rushed, competitive society. Stress, as noted in literature, may be the cause of many health problems. The stress response in humans follows a predictable pattern throughout 24 hours, making it insufficient to obtain a one-time measurement. Multiple assessments are more reliable. While a 24-hour urine cortisol test will give the total cortisol level, it will not determine the pattern throughout the entire 24-hour period. If serum cortisol levels were to be obtained, multiple blood draws would be required for a more accurate assessment, but this is difficult to assess because stress created from drawing blood may cause an artificial elevation of cortisol levels. Therefore, an ideal way to measure free cortisol is through saliva, which is extremely stable. The saliva is conveniently collected at home or at work over a 24-hour period with the first specimen collected in morning (within 30 minutes of arising), the second at noon, the third in late afternoon, and the final specimen collected between 11:00 P.M. to midnight.

The following studies indicate that a saliva hormone study and free hormone in serum is comparable. The Part Study found that women in low stress jobs had lower cortisol one-half hour after waking than women in high stress jobs. Cortisol levels remained the same during the rest of the day. Hellhammer, Wust and Kudleka (2009) state "Salivary cortisol is frequently used as a biomarker of psychological stress." However, psychobiological mechanisms, which trigger the hypothalamus-pituitary-adrenal axis, can only be assessed indirectly by salivary cortisol measures." (p.163) Another study was done on testosterone levels in preadolescent children, that showed testosterone concentration in saliva was comparable to unbound (free or readily available for the body to use) testosterone in serum, Ostatnikova, (2002). Yaneva, (2004) found that "midnight salivary cortisol is an easy and noninvasive means of diagnosing hypercortisolism" (p. 3345). The final study done by Levas and Husebye (2007) recommended saliva cortisol as a first-line screening method for Cushing syndrome and for the improved assessment of adrenal insufficiency (p.730).

The adrenal glands work together with both male and female hormones and the thyroid. If one of the above is not functioning up to par it may affect the other two. Consequently, completing a hormone saliva test may provide additional information in diagnosis. Saliva testing kits are available from a number of labs for evaluating male/ female hormones as well as adrenal hormones in both sexes. Saliva hormone testing measures free hormone or what is available for the body to use. Serum (blood), on the other hand, checks for bound hormone, which is not readily available for the body's use. Consult your healthcare provider to discuss which saliva test should be ordered. Both men and women can be estrogen dominant, meaning they have low progesterone levels. Progesterone is a precursor to many hormones, including male, female and adrenal hormones.

Hair Analysis

The fourth tool for evaluating adrenal stress/fatigue is hair analysis. Published research done as seen on Bio Med Central, *The Lancet, American Journal of Medicine*, and Journal Watch showed a number of studies on the use of hair analysis for detecting drug and alcohol use. The mineral pattern in soft tissue (hair)indicated how well a hormone message was received, and responded to over the last two to three months. However, there must be enough cell receptors with the correct sensitivity to receive this message correctly.

According to Analytical Research Labs (ARL), a biopsy of soft tissue (hair) helps determine the cellular response to hormone signaling regardless of hormone levels. This testing window is two-three months. Hormone abnormalities will show up in a mineral pattern of soft tissue long before hormone levels in blood or saliva change. This test lets a healthcare provider observe and review the interactions of many hormonal and functional systems, and determine how they affect one another. This test may be considered an early stage detection test where which tissue mineral patterns can predict disease trends in healthy individuals.

Since absorption of nutrition takes place at a cellular level rather than at the blood level, whatever nutrients reach the cells is more important than what nutrients appear in the blood. Poor digestion of food prevents those nutrients from being available at the cellular level for use of the cells. In addition to diet, exposure to toxic metals can also cause many diseases and symptoms including fatigue, hypertension, cardiovascular disease, cancer, and diabetes.

The Environmental Protection Agency has approved tissue mineral analysis (hair analysis) for detecting heavy metal poisoning since routine blood tests cannot detect chronic exposure to heavy metals. Some toxic metals are eliminated through the liver, kidney, skin, and hair while those that cannot be eliminated are stored in fatty tissues, joints, hair, and skin. In addition, some toxic metals will replace vital minerals, thus allowing toxic metals to work as a substitute for those when the body is deficient in vital minerals. An example is lead replacing deficient body calcium in the body. Heavy metals can affect the sodium/potassium, levels or the stress ratio, which is a window to adrenal function. If the sodium/potassium levels are inverted—- meaning the potassium levels are higher than the sodium—- the body is in a state of chronic degeneration, and cannot eliminate toxic metals. Individuals with inverse ratio also tend to have low blood sugar, an exhaustion of reserves, decreased immunity, poor digestion, allergic reactions, and adrenal fatigue.

In spite of these previous studies, hair tests can be grossly misunderstood by both natural health practitioners as well as Western medicine practitioners, because of poor research. For example, Drasch and Roider (2002) completed a study on two subjects submitting their hair samples to seven different labs with varying results. Therefore, they concluded hair analysis was not an effective tool for evaluation of nutritional stasis. However, different labs use different methods of hair preparation before testing resulting in different references ranges. According to Analytical Research Labs, washing hair prior to testing rinses out many physiologic minerals in an unpredictable way, but does not change toxic minerals. Most of this information on hair analysis was found on websites of companies doing those tests.

Persons with chronic health or mental health problems, or those with a poor diet may have many nutritional deficiencies. Blood and urine can be examined for organic acids, amino acids, oxidative stress, fatty acids, and toxins. With this information, it can be determined if there are deficiencies in antioxidants, B vitamins, minerals, amino acids, essential fatty acids, or if digestive support is needed. This testing is available through Genova Diagnotics or Great Plains Labs. See your providers for further information.

Another test that has been used for years is called the postural blood pressure test. That information comes from a paper written by Dr. D.C. Ragland, M.D. in 1920. This screening test to evaluate adrenal function is completed by measuring blood pressure from lying to a standing position. The initial blood pressure it taken with the person lying down, then repeated immediately upon standing. The blood pressure should be 4 to 10 mm higher in the standing position than while lying down. If standing blood pressure is lower blood pressure lying down, the adrenals may be hypo-functioning.

CHAPTER 7

Regain Your Energy: The Foundation

Although it may take years, the good news about adrenal stress and fatigue is that individuals can heal with improvements noted all along the way. To begin the healing process, both client and practitioner need to address four areas. These include:

1. Stress modification
2. Balancing the hormone system (including liver/gallbladder detoxification)
3. Blood sugar management
4. Establishing a healthy energy pathway, which includes both diet and healthy digestion.

This chapter will discuss some basic nutritional guidelines that are important for blood sugar handling and the energy pathway. As discussed, there are possibilities of many nutritional deficiencies, and the best way to improve nutrition is through diet. Whether or not adrenal stress or fatigue is present, improving the diet assists anyone in being healthier.

Dr. William Sears, M.D. recommends some basic principles to improve the diet. Wise shoppers check the perimeter of the grocery store, as most healthy foods are found along the outside edges, while the junk foods tend to be in the inner aisles. Secondly, shop for color. The foods with the most color have the greatest amount of phytochemicals. For example choose romaine lettuce or spinach rather than iceberg lettuce, or choose whole grain bread instead of white bread. Thirdly, shop for least processed foods or those closest to nature. Fresh or flash frozen products are best and canned foods are the least nutritious. In summary, eating fewer processed and fast foods, and eating more fruits and vegetables is best.

Whenever possible, select organic produce. Avoid foods with white flour, sugars, fruit juices, sodas and energy drinks. Also, avoid foods containing NutraSweet, Splenda, monosodium glutamate (MSG), hydrolysized vegetable protein, trans-fats, artificial colors, flavors, and preservatives.

Giving the body needed vitamins and minerals from whole food supplements are a second major way of returning to health. Science has discovered over 10,000 nutrients found in food. A simple carrot root has 200 known nutrients and phytonutrients while an apple has 10,000. These nutrients can only be provided by taking vitamin complexes made from whole foods rather than those made in a laboratory. Only vitamins found in nature are groups of chemically related compounds. There is a part of these complexes called organic nutrient. For example, in vitamin C the organic nutrient is ascorbic acid, but this does not include the rest of the vitamin C complex, which includes bioflavonoid complexes, organic copper, F factors, K factors, and J factors. The organic nutrients in vitamin E are the tocopherols (delta, gamma, beta, and alpha tocopherols) but do not include the rest of the E complex (F, F2, E2, E3, xanthine and liposinols). Please see chart below for a picture of whole food vitamin C and E.

There are three types of supplements, one is a true food supplement, and the other two are vitamin supplements or organic nutrient supplements. Whole food supplements are made of raw foods from which the water and fiber has been removed. These supplements are considered natural because they contain all vitamins, enzymes, compounds, and synergistic micronutrients that naturally occur in the raw food. They are processed at a temperature below 112 degree F. in order to preserve enzymes. Two large companies who make "true whole food" based products are Standard Process and NSA, LLC (maker of Juice Plus+).

On the other hand, synthetic vitamins are made by reproducing the organic nutrient in the lab. One example is vitamin C, which is synthesized primarily from corn syrup. While the exact molecular formula

Schematic Representation of
Whole Food Vitamin C and Vitamin E
From <u>The Real Truth About Vitamins & Antioxidants</u>
By Judith DeCava, MS, LNC

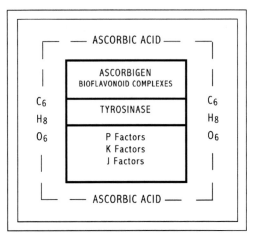

THE FUNCTIONAL ARCHITECTURE
OF VITAMIN C COMPLEX

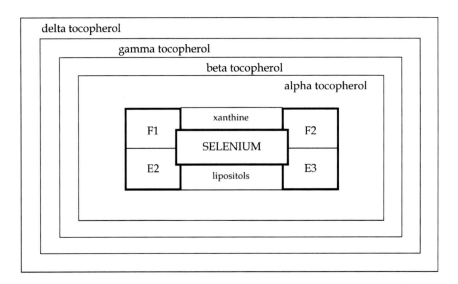

THE FUNCTIONAL ARCHITECTURE OF THE VITAMIN E COMPLEX

of the organic nutrient is replicated in the lab, there are at least two problems with this type of product. These synthetic products contain none of the vital co-factors that are necessary for the body to use the vitamin, or they may not be bioavailable (available for the body to use).

The last type of vitamin is crystalline vitamins or fractionated (not a food supplement). These are made by exposing foods to high-powered chemicals, solvents and heat, which destroy all the co-factors and enzymes, leaving behind only the organic nutrient or individual crystalline vitamin. Like synthetic vitamins, these fractions of the whole nutrient complex lack the co-factors that are so vital for the body to be able to use the vitamin. The positive aspect regarding these vitamins is because it is impossible to remove all the synergistic co-factors from food, so a small amount of these co-factors remain. The question then is, are synthetic and crystalline vitamins effective or non-effective? Are the nutrients in the supplements usable by the body? This usability is known as bioavailability or available to the cells. If co-factors that nature intended to be part of the crystalline vitamin/organic nutrient are not present, or the vitamin is in the wrong configuration (spin) when ingested, then the vitamin is not bioavailable (Robbins 2004).

This author recommends whole food supplements that are made from high quality fruits, vegetables, grains, grasses, and seeds grown in organic or contracted fields which meet high quality standards. The products are harvested when vine-ripe and dried at low heat and then crushed into a powder. The powders are combined, encapsulated, or formed into tablets, thus preserving all the phytochemicals present in the food.

One product I prefer contains vegetable juice powder and pulp from carrot, parsley, beet, kale, broccoli, cabbage, spinach, tomato, gelatin glucomannan, cellulose, calcium ascorbate, calcium carbonate, lactobacillus acidophilus, d-alpha tocopherols, beta- carotene, natural enzyme blend , sugar beet fiber, garlic powder , oat bran, rice bran, mixed tocopherols, dunaliella salina, and folic acid. Compare this with another product (synthetic based supplement) lactose, lecithin, cellulose powder, silicon, choline chloride, methionine, alpha- tocopherol, inositol, magnesium stearate, torula dried yeast, calcium, zinc, thiamine, riboflavin, vitamin A, pyridoxine hydrochloride, vitamin B12. In the first example, vitamins and nutrients are derived mainly from recognizable food sources; in the second brand vitamins and nutrients are manufactured, chemical isolates that are not recognized as food sources.

With supplements, more is not always better. Food naturally contains small quantities of nutrients and phytochemicals that work together. When choosing supplements, consider where the raw ingredients come from. Are they grown on company farms or are they imported from China? What kind of testing is done on the products? The best advice is to find a qualified healthcare provider who can work with you to recommend the best supplements for your needs.

Besides the diet, the energy pathway also includes digestion. Many people think that too much acid causes indigestion; however, indigestion is actually caused by too little acid. Poorly digested food sits in the stomach and rots. This rotting food produces acids, which then causes reflux. Suggestions for improving digestion include:

- ❖ Drink liquids 30 to 45 minutes before the meal and drinking only sips during the meal. Wait 1 to 2 hours after the meal to drink more liquids. Drinking too many fluids during the meal further dilutes digestive enzymes.
- ❖ Eat food slowly, chew it well.
- ❖ Try food combining. Eat fruits by themselves; vegetables and starch together, or meat and starch together. Different foods require different digestive enzymes, thus using food combining can improve digestion.
- ❖ Follow a gluten free diet. Many gluten sensitive people have increased reflux when foods containing gluten are eaten.
- ❖ Take a digestive enzyme such as Multizyme ® or Enzycore ® from Standard Process.
- ❖ If antacids or H-2 blockers such as Prilosec (purple pills) are taken, gradually wean off them while following the above recommendations. Stopping these medications abruptly can cause a rebound of excessive acid production. It is important to discontinue these medications because they prevent absorption of important nutrients—especially minerals and trace minerals leading to nutritional deficiencies, which can cause osteoporosis and cardiovascular disease.
- ❖ To enhance healing of the gastrointestinal (GI) tract take products that include deglycyrrhizinated licorice (will not affect

blood pressure), marshmallow, or Slippery Elm, colostrum, okra, or digestive enzyme containing L-glutamine.

Another area to address in the healing process is blood sugar handling. Individuals with adrenal stress and fatigue crave simple carbohydrates and stimulants such as soda, coffee, or sweets in order to give them more energy. This causes highs and lows in blood sugar and insulin that can increase weight and fatigue. In order to correct this condition, eat six small meals daily or three meals and three snacks.

Foods that moderate blood sugar are nuts, apple or celery with peanut butter, cheese, vegetables, eggs, tuna or chicken salad, green salad with cheese or chicken. Replace crackers with cucumbers, and scrambled eggs with spinach. Follow a low carbohydrate, or Mediterranean- type diet. Avoid foods made with white sugar and white flour, junk foods (foods with little or no nutritional value), fast foods, cookies, and candy. Begin weaning yourself from coffee and soda by replacing these with water and green or white teas. The goal of this is to maintain even blood sugar and insulin levels throughout the day because highs and lows in blood sugar further stress the adrenals. Supplements that can help with blood sugar handling are Diaplex® 2 at each meal, Cataplex GTF® (contains chromium), zinc, Magnesium lactate (increase insulin sensitivity) and Gymnema (take one 2 to 3 times daily). See a health care provider who has current nutritional experience for further guidance.

Balancing hormones and detoxification is a third area to address for achieving healing. Both males and females with adrenal stress and fatigue may have estrogen dominance or low levels of progesterone. Progesterone is a steroid hormone and is used by the body to produce cortisol and other adrenal hormones. Estrogen dominance can be identified from the Systems Survey, patient observation, or saliva testing. Support of the liver/gall bladder can help the body eliminate extra estrogen. An excellent supplement to use before a gallbladder cleanse is A-F BetaFood® from Standard Process. There are a number of different suggestions for gallbladder cleanses. One suggestion is drinking 4 ounces of apple juice every ½ hour for 12 hours. No food should be eaten during this time but plenty of water is allowed. After twelve hours, drink 4 ounces of warmed, extra virgin olive oil. You will cleanse sometime within the next 24 hours. (Caution is advised for diabetics as apple juice can raise blood sugar.) Lastly, consider a detoxification program. There are a number of different programs available, one is the Purification Program from Standard Process. The Purification Program, besides detoxifying the body, will also lower triglycerides and cholesterol.

The last area to discuss in this book section is stress modification because it plays a major role in adrenal stress and fatigue. Stress is not just what is happening today but also what has occurred over a lifetime. The Holmes-Rahe Life Stress Inventory has been used for years to evaluate stress levels since it was published in the *Journal* of *Psychosomatic Research* in 1967.

Life Event	Mean Value
1. Death of spouse	100
2. Divorce	73
3. Marital separation from mate	65
4. Detention in jail or other institution	63
5. Death of a close family member	63
6. Major personal injury or illness	53
7. Marriage	50
8. Being fired from work	47
9. Marital reconciliation with mate	45
10. Retirement from work	45
11. Major change in the health or behavior of a family member	44
12. Pregnancy	40
13. Sexual difficulties	39
14. Major Business readjustment	39
15. Gaining a new family member (birth, adoption, older adult moving in)	39
16. Major change in financial state	38
17. Death of a close friend	37
18. Change to a different line of work	36
19. Major change in number of arguments with spouse	35
20. Taking on a mortgage (home or business)	31
21. Foreclosure on mortgage or loan	30
22. Major change in responsibilities at work	29
23. Child leaving home	29
24. In-law troubles	29

25. Outstanding personal achievement 28
26. Spouse beginning or ceasing work outside home..................26
27. Beginning or ceasing formal schooling 26
28. Major change in living conditions (new home,
    remodeling) 25
29. Change in personal habits 24
30. Troubles with boss 23
31. Change in working hours or conditions 20
32. Changes in residence..20
33. Change in school 20
34. Major change in usual type or amount of recreation..............19
35. Major change in church activity..................................18
36. Major change in social activities 17
37. Taking on a loan (car, furniture)................................16
38. Major change in sleeping habits (more or less) 16
39. Major change in family get togethers 15
40. Major change in eating habits 15
41. Vacation..13
42. Major holiday 12
43. Minor violation of the law 11

In this test, the client adds up the point value for all factors occurring within the last year. A score of 150 points or less means you have a relatively low stress level related to life changes and a low susceptibility of health issues caused by stress. 150-300 points implies about a 50% chance of a major health concern within the next two years while 300 points or more raises these odds to about 80%, according to the Holmes-Rahe statistical prediction model. Bear in mind, however, that this information was written in 1967. Today's life is busier than ever and the nutritional status of Americans has decreased, so factors increasing stress are higher.

To heal from adrenal stress and fatigue necessitates making life-style changes. Pace yourself, and avoid pushing yourself to exhaustion. Be kind to yourself by allowing some personal time weekly. Avoid people who steal your energy. Go to bed early enough, or sleep late enough, to get at least eight hours of sleep. Become informed about your health care. Find things that make you laugh. Do activities you enjoy rather than pushing yourself to exhaustion. Start a mild to moderate exercise program. Avoid being critical and harsh with yourself. Lastly, find an inner balance and sense of peace.

Another way to reduce stress is Neurolinguistic Programming (NLP) in which a person learns to alter their perceptions of an event. This is called reframing or seeing a situation from a different view.

Any sort of relaxation reduces stress. There many ways to enhance the relaxation response, such as deep breathing, vacations, yoga, meditation, sleep, exercise, music therapy, acupuncture, massage, chiropractic care, and others. Because busy jobs and family schedules often leave spouses going in different directions, in addition to planning some "me time," consider setting some time aside for just you and your spouse or partner at least once a month.

Summary

After completing this research, it appears adrenal stress and fatigue is indeed a real condition with the underlying causes being stress, poor nutritional choices, and lifestyle choices. Considering this information, it is evident that education is important for all ages regarding dietary and life-style choices. Individuals making better choices regarding life style and nutrition can prevent many health care issues including adrenal stress/fatigue.

PART TWO:

TO THE HEALTHCARE PROVIDER

CHAPTER 8

Healing Adrenals with Nutritional Supplements

THERE ARE A number of vitamins required for the adrenals to function properly. The most important of these is vitamin C. As the level of cortisol increases, so does the need for vitamin C, which acts as an antioxidant for the adrenal cortex. A study conducted on adrenal weights in rats exposed to cold stress showed that ascorbic acid was concentrated in the adrenals of the rats (Woods, 1957). Another study, conducted by Payayatty, (2007), showed "Adrenocorticotrophic hormone stimulation increases adrenal vein, but not peripheral vein vitamin C concentrations. This data is the first study in humans showing that hormone-regulated vitamin secretion occurs and that adrenal vitamin C paracrine secretion is part of the stress response. Tight control of peripheral vitamin C concentration is permissive of higher local concentrations that may have paracrine functions" (p. 145). Humans must consume vitamin C, as they are unable to convert blood glucose into vitamin C like most animals do. As discussed previously, providing clients with whole-food vitamin C as in Standard Process Cataplex C®, or Juice Plus+® Orchard Blend provides the whole food complex which contains ascorbic acid, bioflavonoid complexes, organic copper (tyrosinase), F, K, and J factors. Each 15 mg of whole-food vitamin C is equal to 1500 mg of ascorbic acid.

Another necessary nutrient family is—-the B vitamins—- including pantothenic acid, niacin, vitamin B6, and B12 are also needed for healthy adrenal glands. Pantothenic acid, or vitamin B5, is a necessary part of coenzyme A (CoA). This assists in converting glucose into energy by metabolizing carbohydrates, proteins, and fats. This also influences hormones and cholesterol (Wilson, J., 2001). Foods rich in vitamin B5 include meats, liver, kidney, fish, chicken, vegetables, legumes, yeast, eggs, and milk. This deficiency is rare. According to Medline Plus, vitamin B5 is rated C, or unclear scientific evidence, for use in athletic performance, ADHD, burns, high cholesterol, osteoarthritis, rheumatoid arthritis, wound healing and radiation, and skin irritations, however, there was no mention of use for adrenal stress/fatigue regarding adrenals (U.S. National Library of Medicine, National Institute of Health, 2006b).

Large amounts of niacin, or vitamin B3, are necessary for the molecular structure of several coenzymes that are used in adrenal hormones. Niacin, according is used to assist the body in lowering high cholesterol, healing atherosclerosis, helping prevent of second heart attacks, and for possible use in those with Alzheimer's disease and osteoarthritis. In theory, individuals with acne, macular degeneration, alcohol dependence, anti-aging, anxiety, Bell's palsy, high blood pressure, hypothyroidism, schizophrenia, migraine headache, and multiple scleroses have used niacin supplementation. (US National Library of Medicine, National Institute of Health, 2006b). Whole food niacin is available from Standard Process in Drenamin® (contains Cataplex®G).

Adrenal cell extracts provide nourishment and assist the adrenal glands to rebuild themselves so they can again produce the needed hormones to function. Natural or synthetic steroids such as cortisone, prednisone, and prednisolone suppress the adrenal glands. This in turn interferes with the normal feedback loops that assist in regulating adrenal hormones and delay or prevent healing (Wilson J., 2001). On the other hand, Cataplex® B and Cataplex® G—both from Standard Process are good choices because they make up the whole food B complex. Vitamin B12 is available in Cataplex B12® or Folic acid B12®.

Dr. Royal Lee chose to call vitamins complexes or cataplex (cata in Greek means concentrate and plexa means many) rather than vitamin B or vitamin C. Dr. Lee divided the B vitamins into two different products which are used differently. When using Cataplex® B or G consider the following information: Use Cataplex® B to support the body when symptoms of inability to metabolize lactic acid are present such as muscle weakness, lack of stamina, drowsiness after eating, and muscular soreness. Motor nerve conductivity and nerve integrity with symptoms of rapid heartbeat, hyperirritability, a feeling of band being the around head, melancholia or feelings of sadness, are other indications for Cataplex® B. The last two indications for using Cataplex® B are when vasodilatation, due to lactic acid excess, is present (as in swelling of ankles and diminished urination) and when there is a craving for sweets. Cataplex® G, on the other hand, should be used to support the body if symptoms of muscle spasms, blurred vision, and loss of muscular control, numbness, night sweats, rapid digestion, or sensitivity to noise are present. Cataplex® G is also indicated when there is redness in the palms of the hands and the bottom of feet, visible veins on the chest and abdomen, and hemorrhoids from edema secondary to liver disease. Pellagra–type symptoms, such as apprehension, nervousness that cause loss of appetite or indigestion and gastritis, are further indications for Cataplex® G. Finally, forgetfulness or thinning hair from vasoconstriction are additional indications for Cataplex® G. Use more Cataplex® G than B when blood pressure is high or more Cataplex® B than G when blood pressure is low.

Other supplements that can be used to support the adrenals are glandulars, which supply the raw materials to assist the adrenal glands in healing. One such product is Whole Dessicated Adrenal®, which should only be used short-term to give the adrenals a boost. On the other hand, Drenamin®, which contains Drenatrophin PMG®, CataplexC®, and Cataplex G®, can be used long-term to assist in healing the adrenals.

Individuals with adrenal fatigue often have mitochonical dysfunction. According to a study conducted by Teitelbaum, D-ribose reduced significantly the clinical symptoms in patients suffering from fibromyalgia and chronic fatigue. (D-ribose, a five-carbon sugar, is required to provide the building blocks for ATP, which provides energy within each cell.) In addition to chronic fatigue, research has shown that conditions such as congestive heart failure, chronic ischemic heart disease, post open-heart surgery, or myocardial infarction, mitochondrial dysfunction can also benefit from D-ribose.

PS (Phosphorylated Serine) is found in higher amounts in brain cells and is shown to help and restore the hippocampus. It also helps to decrease high cortisol levels, and helps relieve the resulting insomnia, anxiety, and stress caused by high cortisol levels. Nerozzi his study on cortisol states that there are a number of alterations detected in the HPA axis in normal elderly subjects, abnormal elevations of basal morning cortisol values in three subjects; disruption of the circadian cortisol pattern noted in four subjects; and early cortisol escape phenomenon in seven subjects. Two subjects had a true non-suppression. Thus, early cortisol escape phenomenon appears to be a consistent abnormality in all subjects (Nerozzi, 1989). This information supports the use of Phosphorylated Serine when high cortisol is present.

In summary, this chapter discusses basic information on supplement use for the provider to consider in assisting his patients on the path of healing. See the appendix for a summary of possible supplements to use.

CHAPTER 9

Healing Adrenals with Herbal Products

IN THIS CHAPTER we will discuss common herbs used to assist in healing the adrenals. There are a number of herbs on the market leaving the patient at loss over which one to pick. The FDA sets no standard for herbal companies. Cost and quality vary widely. Reputable companies must work with herbs on a regular basis and know that plant quality depends on growing location, soil quality, harvesting, drying, and storage methods of the raw product. Quality begins when the company examines the plant before purchasing. Plants should be checked for color, aroma, texture, content of active ingredients, microbial levels, pesticides or herbicides, heavy metals, and radiation exposure. Other important tests include looking for possible substitution of species, adulteration of the herb, quality of the raw product, and quality of extraction. A high quality method of extraction is 1:2 cold percolations where no heat or concentration is used which may damage the plant. High Performance Liquid Chromatography (HPLC) is a testing method used by many companies to check the active ingredients.

Since most individuals will not spend time investigating the quality of herbal products, seeking the advice of a qualified health care provider who routinely uses herbal products is recommended. One such company that meets all the above requirements is MediHerb, a popular herbal company of healthcare professionals in Australia. MediHerb has been available in the United States since 2001 through a partnership with Standard Process.

The following herbal products have been found helpful in assisting the body to cope with stress and healing of the adrenal glands. The dosages discussed are recommended dosages from literature written by Kerry Bone, co-founder of MediHerb, Head of Research and Development of Medi-Herb, and Principal of the Australian College of Phytotherapy.

The first herb, Eleuthero (Siberian Ginseng), an adaptogen, assists the body to cope with stress, supports the immune system, and increases vitality. It is available for ingestion as a root decoction, liquid extract, tablets, or as a powered herb. The typical dosage is from 1-4 grams daily or 2-8 ml a day for 1:2 extract. For healthy individuals, it can be used for six weeks followed by a two-week break. However, the German Commission E recommends no more than three months of continual use before taking a break and using it again. There are no side effects expected if used as directed. According to Bone (2000), Eleuthero should be discontinued during any infection and should not be used in individuals with extremely high blood pressure. It should be noted that there are a number of animal and human studies showing "improved performance and increased stamina" with increased mental and physical ability when using Eleuthero. In addition, this herb has also been used by individuals in China and Russia for conditions affecting the heart, kidneys, and nervous system. There are no known interactions noted between Eleuthero and medications. A study on twenty elderly patients showed that Eleuthero "improves mental health and social functioning after four weeks of therapy, although these differences attenuate with continued use"(Cicero, 2004).

The second herb, another adaptogenic herb, Ashwaganda (Witha-nia) has been used by Ayurvedic medicine practitioners to support the body for disability and premature aging. It functions as a tonic, normalizes the immune system, is a mild sedative, and is an anti-inflammatory. Ashwaganda supports individuals with asthma, bronchitis, arthritis, dementia, exhaustion (especially from stress), to assist in recovery after a long illness, and for a depressed white cell count. Dosage is 3-6 grams daily of dried root by decoction or 6-12 ml of 1:2 liquid extract per day. Researchers studying Ashwaganda (in 101 healthy males aged 50 to 59) found an increase in hemoglobin, less graying of hair, decrease in nail calcium and serum cholesterol, and improvement in sexual performance. There are no known contraindications, interactions with medications, or side effects to Ashwaganda (Bone, Mills, 2000).

Practitioners have used the third herb, the root of Rehmannia, for support in autoimmune diseases, allergies, and aiding in healing the adrenal cortex. Rehmannia may also protect the adrenals against the suppressive effect of steroids and chemotherapy. It is safe to use for individuals with hypertension (Bone, Mills, 2000). A study conducted in July 2007 showed Rehmannia significantly improved insulin resistance of Hep G2 cells induced by high insulin (Guo, 2007). Rehmannia is an antipyretic, adrenal restorative, anti-hemorrhage, anti-inflammatory, mild laxative, and is ideal for low DHEA-S and elevated cortisol. Rehmannia, unlike some herbs, may be used long term with no expected adverse effects or interactions at the dosage of 10-30 grams per day of dried root or 4-12 ml daily of 1:2 liquid extract (Bone, Mills, 2000).

The fourth herb, licorice, has a long history of use in ancient China, Egypt, and Greece, as well as Western herbal medicine. It decreases inflammation of the upper digestive tract, increases anti-inflammatory effects of glucocorticords, potentates cortisol and increases movement of mucus from the respiratory tract. "Licorice is anti-inflammatory, mucoprotective, adrenal tonic, expectant, demulcent, mild laxative and anti-carcinogenic" (Bone, Mills, 2000) and (U.S. National Library of Medicine, 2006). Therapeutic uses of this herb include supporting persons with bronchitis, cough, ulcers, gastritis, adrenal insufficiency, Addison's disease, and inflammation of the urinary tract. Other uses include support for steroid dependency and as a flavoring for unpleasant medicines. Dosages range from 2-6 ml of 1:1 liquid extract. The German Commission E states that licorice should not be taken longer than six to eight weeks at higher doses. In addition, the German Commission E cautions its use by those clients with a history of hypertension, even when the hypertension is controlled with medication. A high potassium intake will decrease the risk of the Aldosterone-like side effect. Deglycyrrhizinized licorice does not carry the cautions regarding hypertension that glycyrrhizinized licorice does; however, it may stimulate the adrenal glands causing difficulty sleeping. Care should be taken not to give multiple products that contain licorice without careful monitoring.

Two compounds found in licorice, GL (glycyrrhizin acid) and GA (glycyrrhetinic acid), change the metabolism of steroid hormones. GL increases the effect of cortisone by slowing down the metabolism of corticosteroids. It increases the anti-inflammatory effect of cortisol while suppressing ACTH synthesis and secretion. This effect can be used to an advantage when weaning someone from steroidal anti-inflammatory drugs. GA antagonizes the effect of orally administered estrogen, not estrogen produced in the body. GA slows the enzyme that inactivates cortisol and can cause sodium retention (Bone, Mills, 2000). This above information makes licorice an option when supporting a client with adrenal fatigue. Licorice and Rehmannia are combined in a product called Adrenal Complex from MediHerb.

The fifth herb, Tribulus, increases testosterone and fertility in men, as well as increasing energy and stamina (Brown, 2000). Tribulus also appears to increase Follicle-Stimulating Hormone (FSH) in pre-menopausal women, in turn which increases levels of estradiol and estrogen dominance. In postmenopausal women, Tribulus acts by binding with vacant receptors in the hypothalamus and may convince the body there is more estrogen than is actually present. A similar action in men is present via the hypothalamus but Leuteinizing Hormone (LH) is increased (Hywood, 2004).

The sixth herb, Korean Ginseng (Panex), is a valued herbal plant used frequently in Chinese Medicine. According to the Chinese, Panex restores vital energy, increases production of vital fluids, and encourages health and length of life. The list of actions of Panex includes adaptogenic, tonic, immunomodulator, cardiotonic and cancer preventive. It is dosed at 1-10 grams daily of the dried root for up to three months (Bone, Mills, 2000). Since ginseng acts mainly on the hypothalamus, with some action on the adrenal cortex through the anterior pituitary and ACTH release, it is an optional supplement for adrenal stress/fatigue. The quality of Panex is a concern. A study published in the U.S.A. in 1978 showed a wide variety in the quality of several products showing no detectable ginsenosides in their product (Liberti, 1978). Standardized extract of ginseng mixed with vitamins and minerals and 5:1 extract of ginsenoside has been used in over 60 published clinical studies. Panex may be too stimulating for some individuals (Bone, Mills, 2000).

The seventh herb, Rhodiola (Rhodiola Rosea, Roseroot, and Golden Root) is a plant that grows in cold areas around the world, such as in much of the Arctic Asian Mountains, Rocky Mountains, and European mountains. Common uses for this herb are to support memory, attention span, mental sharpness, anxiety/panic attacks, depression, mental/physical fatigue, and focus. In Russia, Rhodiola has also been used to improve both mental and physical performance, fatigue, and sickness resulting from high altitudes. The Russian's have used Rhodiola for hundreds of years to cope with the harsh Siberian climates and stressful lifestyle. Rhodiola is an adaptogen, which increases the body's resistance to a wide range of stressors, whether chemical, physical, or biological. While the exact of action is unknown, both clinical and lab research show that Rhodiola affects and promotes healthy neurotransmitter balance in the brain and provides some relief for depressed mood, mild to moderate mood changes, and physical/mental fatigue, as well as occasional anxiety and panic attacks. There are very few side effects noted with Rhodiola's use suggesting that it has a low toxicity. MediHerb combines Rhodiola and Ginseng at the dosage of 1 to 2 tabs 2 times daily.

Since many individuals with adrenal fatigue also have a poor immune system, the last herb to discuss is Astragalus. Astragalus has been used for hundreds of years in traditional Chinese Medicine to restore and strengthen the immune response and increase vitality. Clinical trials have shown impaired immune systems, associated with low white count in cancer treatments, viral infections, and following herpes simplex infection, have all responded to Astragalus. Dosage is 10-30g daily or 4-8 ml daily of 1:2 liquid extract. It may be taken long-term except during an acute infection (Bone, Mills, 2000).

Finally, one of the main symptoms of individuals with adrenal stress and fatigue is carbohydrate craving. When completing a diet history, those individuals often indicate that they drink many caffeinated sodas for energy, as well as eating snacks and sweets. In order to heal, carbohydrate craving must be controlled. Gymnema is a woody plant grown in the tropical forests of central and southern India. It has been used in Ayurvedic medicine for centuries to support individuals with diabetes. The flowers, leaves, and fruits of this plant support persons with high or low blood pressure, rapid heartbeat and irregular heart rhythm. Chewing these leaves or taking the liquid extract destroys the ability to taste sweet. One study showed a reduction of cholesterol and triglycerides in diabetic patients. Another study showed the reduction in weight and upper abdominal, waist, and hip circumferences in individuals taking supplements with Gymnema. Dosage of Gymnema leaf 10:1 extract is 400 mg 1-2 times daily.

CHAPTER 10

Healing Adrenals with Protomorphogen Extracts, Animal Tissue Extracts, and Concentrates

PROTOMORPHOGEN EXTRACTS, ANIMAL tissue extracts, along with concentrates have a role in assisting the body to heal from adrenal stress and fatigue. Glandulars are made from whole organs that are dried at low temperature, ground up and placed in capsules. These desiccated products contain all components of the gland including functional and connective tissues. They are not glandular replacements, however, like any healthy tissue; they are used to supply nutritional support. In addition, they provide both known and unknown factors which are found in and required by healthy tissue. Desiccated products are available in a number of Standard Process products such as Adrenal *Desiccated* and Spleen *Desiccated* and should only be used for 30 to 90 days. (Kincaid, 2004).

Cytosol extracts are aqueous or enzymatic extracts of precursors to active metabolic forms from certain active endocrine tissues such as Adrenal Cytosol Extract and Orchex®. These will not promote tissue rebuilding, but rather will assist in the day-to-day function of a system that is operating at suboptimal level by supplying certain nutritional factors that the body can immediately use, because Cytosol **TM** extracts work quickly. (Kincaid, 2004).

According to Dr. Royal Lee, Protomorphogen Extracts are "single cells of every organ in the body have their own specific types of these cell determinants which carry the blueprints of the whole organ." They act like homeopathics that promote healing over time. Dr. Royal Lee commented on the work by Alexia Carrel: "It has been demonstrated that one kind of cell may be reconstructed to become another kind of cell. Liver cells can be cultured in a flask and put in some connective tissue from the kidney and soon you will have kidney cells instead of liver cells." Part of Dr. Royal Lee's protomorphology theory states that by changing the concentration of the blueprint material in culture medium, the basic tissue will follow the pattern being set up by the blueprint material

Dr. Royal Lee published a book on protomorphogens in 1947 and began releasing his products in the early 1950's. He felt that disease was caused by internal breakdown resulting from poor nutrition. Examples of this would be children with frequent colds, strep or yeast infection, or adults with complaints of fatigue or fibromyalgia. He noted it takes time to heal—for each year the problem has been present, a minimum of one month is required to begin healing. Dr. Lee taught that:

- ❖ All cells secrete, as a product of their metabolism a relatively stable substance (PMG).
- ❖ Dilute amounts of this substance must be present in media for initial cell division to occur.
- ❖ Accumulation of substance in media inhibits mitosis in proportion to its concentration; too much results in lysis (gradual disappearance of symptoms of an acute disease with recovery) of inhibits.
- ❖ There is a relationship between the concentration of PMGs in protoplasm and media, which explains the lag period and S-curve.
- ❖ Controlling factor is concentration of PMGs in cells that is continually produced.
- ❖ PMGs as found in living organisms lead to protein for building neuro protein

In summary PMGs stimulate normal growth. In a weakened body, it promotes to normal healing. In autoimmune disease, there are too many antibodies, which attack various organs. Introducing a supplement containing PMGs acts as a decoy so the gland may heal, however, since PMGs are not glandular, the response is slow. The greater the need for a PMG the greater the likelihood a histamine response may occur, so advise the client to begin slowly and advance dosage as tolerated.

CHAPTER 11

Dissertation Design

Introduction

The purpose of this author's study was to gather evidence to document the extent of adrenal stress and fatigue in a selected adult population. The independent variable, lifestyle, included diet, supplementation, and lifestyle changes. Adrenal stress and fatigue, the dependent variable, was defined either by answers to specific questions from a validated questionnaire or through medical history obtained from the survey. The study presented evidence of: 1) a direct association between poor nutrition and adrenal stress and fatigue and 2) a direct association between improved nutrition and adrenal stress and fatigue.

Methodology

A survey was e-mailed to an existing list of this author's clients and customers of Organic Ways Health Food Store in order to evaluate the number of persons who may have had symptoms of adrenal stress/fatigue. The survey included questions regarding basic personal information, medical and diet history, current health symptoms, and lifestyle questions. This researcher gathered survey evaluations and treatments done by both Western and natural health practitioners. Data was gathered using a survey to investigate the relationship between nutrition, lifestyle, and adrenal fatigue for adults age 18 to 75. The survey included questions regarding diet, supplement use, lifestyle factors, and questions looking for signs of adrenal stress/fatigue. The survey data was then analyzed to determine the extent of the relationships between nutrition, lifestyle, and adrenal stress/fatigue in the sample group.

Survey Analysis Plan

All questions on this survey were evaluated together or on their own. The three survey guidelines included Lifestyles Guide, Nutrition Guide, and the Endocrine Guide, which included thyroid, pituitary, and adrenal. In addition, blood sugar handling, digestion, liver/gallbladder, and B complex deficiency were included in the Endocrine Guid, because these have a huge bearing on the health of the endocrine system. Please see Appendix A for the survey questions. The following information will describe the survey tool.

General Information

Question 1 (height and weight) was used to determine Body Mass Index which is an evaluation of healthy weight to height. According to the National Institute of Health, those with a BMI of 19-24 were within the normal weight range; those with a BMI of 25-29 were considered overweight; those with a BMI of 30-39 were considered obese, and those with a BMI of 40-54 were considered extremely obese. This information was used to answer research questions regarding the average weight of those with adrenal stress/fatigue.

Question 2 (respondent's age) was used to determine the average age of those with adrenal stress/fatigue and addressed research question 11. The respondents were grouped in categories: 20-29, 30-39, 40-49, 50-59, 60-69, and 70-79 years of age.

Question 4 and 5 were for general demographic information and not designed to answer any research question.

Nutritional Guide

Questions 1 to 10 under the nutritional information formed the nutritional guide. Question 1 in the diet and nutrition section addressed frequency of eating out. The nutritional guide was an important part of the survey as it showed those with a poorer diet had increased symptoms of adrenal stress/fatigue.

Most of the questions in the nutritional guide had a maximum score of five points per question. Please see Appendix A for the Survey with Scoring for more information on each question. The maximum score was 80 for the nutrition guide. A "very healthy diet" was 70 to 80 points. A score of 60 to 69 was considered a "healthy diet" and any score from 50 to 59 was considered an "unhealthy diet." A score less than 50 was considered a "very unhealthy diet."

Questions 1 and 2 in the nutrition section had a maximum score of 5 with a healthy score being 4. Question 3 had a maximum score of 20, with healthy being 15. Questions 4 and 5 had a maximum score of 25, with healthy being 20. Question 6 had a maximum score of 28, with healthy being 20. Question 7 had maximum score of 15, with healthy being 12. Question 8 about the type of diet, was used to see if there was a relationship between diet, the nutrition guide, and adrenal stress/fatigue.

Lifestyle Questions

The Lifestyle Guide consisted of questions 1 through 8, and was used to assist in analyzing lifestyle and its relationship to adrenal stress/fatigue. The maximum score was 25 points with a healthy lifestyle being 25 to 16 points. A score of 15 or less was considered an unhealthy lifestyle. Each question was worth five points. Questions 1, 2, and 3 were combined to evaluate sleep patterns. The maximum score was 4 with healthy being 3 and an unhealthy score being 2 or less. Question 2 was important in evaluating adrenal stress/fatigue, as those individuals often had a "second wind" in the evening and had difficulty getting to sleep. In addition, they tended to be slow-starters in the morning and slept later. Question 5 regarding exercise had a maximum score of 5, with 4 being healthy and less than 2 unhealthy. Question 6 regarding use of tobacco had a score of 5 as healthy for those that did not use tobacco, and 0 as unhealthy for those that did use tobacco. Question 7 regarding alcohol use had a maximum score of 5 with 5 being healthy. Those that drank alcohol daily were considered unhealthy. Question 8 evaluated water intake with a maximum score of 5 being healthy and a score of less than 4 being unhealthy. Lastly, Question 9 evaluated diagnosed health conditions and medications taken for these conditions.

Endocrine Guide

The last section of the survey evaluated conditions often seen with individuals having adrenal stress/fatigue. Group A, B, C, D, E, F, G, H, I, and J were included in this guide. Each indication was scored according to severity with A being mild or once or twice a month, B being moderate or weekly, and C being severe or daily. Each indication noted received 1 point for an A, 2 points for a B, and 3 points for a C. Group A represented blood sugar handling. The higher score indicated a greater chance the individual had problems with low blood sugar.

Group B evaluated liver/gallbladder and Group C evaluated digestion. When assisting individuals to improve their health, digestion, including liver/gallbladder functions, must be supported or repaired. If an individual is not digesting well, it is wise to consider placing him on a gluten-free diet to enhance absorption of needed healing nutrients.

Group D and E indications were associated with hyperthyroid (Group D) and hypothyroid (Group E). The higher score in each group was indicative of thyroid issues. Many individuals with adrenal stress and fatigue had indications of thyroid problems. Group F (hyperpituitary) and Group G (hypopituitary) evaluated for indications associated with pituitary problems. The higher score of this group indicated a greater chance of HPA axis disregulation. Group H (hyperactive adrenal or adrenal stress) and Group I (hypoactive adrenal or adrenal fatigue) dealt with the probability of adrenal stress and fatigue. The higher scores in Group H and I showed a greater chance of adrenal stress and fatigue. Finally, Group J evaluated for indications of B complex deficiency. B vitamins are needed at the cellular level to process fats, carbohydrates, and protein, and to support the adrenals' ability to handle stress.

CHAPTER 12

Study Design and Results

Introduction

THE PUBLIC IS just beginning to be aware of the relationship of diet and health to disease. In this study, it was noted that those with a diet higher in simple carbohydrates and junk foods had more health problems including adrenal stress/fatigue. Individuals with adrenal stress and fatigue craved more simple carbohydrates and caffeinated beverages to give them energy. Blood sugars often went from highs to lows resulting in fatigue and hypoglycemia. The survey also showed those with the lowest intake of fruits and vegetables had more health problems including adrenal stress and fatigue.

Analysis of Data

One hundred and five surveys were completed. Twenty-one of those surveyed completed an Adrenal Stress Index test along with blood sugar, blood count, and thyroid studies to rule out other causes of fatigue. Six of the individuals did not complete diet and lifestyle questions, but did answer questions on symptoms they were experiencing. These surveys were also included in the data. When the data was evaluated, consideration was given to the self-reporting nature of the survey as well as the possibility of underreported diet history and symptoms.

Survey Demographics

The respondents reflected the demographics of the population in this author's community, which was Caucasian (100%). However, the survey was not limited to any group intentionally. The majority of the respondents were from Iowa (88.5%); other states represented included Nebraska (7.6%), Kansas (.095%), New York (.095%), Colorado (.095%), and Indiana (.095%). (See Appendix B, Chart B2)

The BMI (body mass index) was calculated using the information on height and weight. Weights ranged from 101 to 315 while height ranged from 60 to 71 inches. BMIs ranged from 17.8 to 46.8 with the average being 28.5. Those individuals with a BMI of less than 18.5 were considered underweight, those with BMI 18.5 to 24.9 were considered normal weight, those with BMI 25 to 29.9 were considered overweight, and those whose BMI was 30 or greater were considered obese. On the average, respondents were in the overweight range. It is this researcher's observation that those with adrenal stress and fatigue tend to make poorer choices in food which possibly relates to their higher weights. In addition, when individuals had adrenal stress and fatigue, they had more difficulty processing fats, carbohydrates, and protein because of nutritional deficiencies such as B vitamins and gallbladder symptoms. They also tended to crave simple carbohydrates, which caused higher insulin levels and weight gain.

The respondents' ages ranged between 19 and 79, with an average age of 49. The majority of the respondents were between ages 50 and 69 years old (55.7%). The age range of all respondents was: 19 to 29 years old (5.8%), 30 to 39 years old (15.4%), 40 to 49 years old (13.5%), 50 to 59 years old (38.5%), 60 to 69 years old (17.3%), and 70 to 79 years old (9.6%).

Diet and Nutrition

Of the 105 surveys returned, four did not complete the nutrition guide. Seven (7%) did not eat out weekly. Eighty-two (82%) respondents ate out one to three times a week. Therefore, 89 (89%) scored as being healthy. Ten (10%) ate out four to six times a week, four (4%) ate out seven to ten times a week, and none ate out greater than ten times weekly. (See Appendix B Chart B5)

The subjects' beverages included in the nutrition guide were water, coffee, teas (herbal, green, and black), soft drinks, water, milk (whole, skim, 1% and 2%), soy and almond beverages. Thirty-nine (36.8%) scored a maximum score of 5, while 30 (28%) scored 4, meaning 69 (65%) choose healthy beverages. 37 of the respondents (35%) choose less healthy beverages. Ninety-six (90.5%) drank water, 49 (46%) drank coffee, 1 (.94%) drank decaffeinated coffee, 27 (25%) drank black tea while 9 (8.4%) drank green tea, 24 (22%) drank 1 or more sodas daily, with 10 (9.4%) choosing diet sodas. Lastly, 21 (19.8%) drank milk and 1 (.94%) drank soy beverage daily.

All respondents on the survey consumed vegetables at least weekly. Seven (7%) consumed vegetables one to three times a week, while seventeen (17%) consumed them four to six times weekly. Fifteen (15%) consumed a vegetable daily, while forty-four (44%) consumed two to three vegetables daily. Ten (10%) consumed four to five servings of vegetables daily. Only five (5%) consumed six or more servings of vegetables daily.

The consummation of fruit varied with respondents. Two (2%) did not eat any fruit weekly, while one (1%) consumed one fruit weekly. Twenty-one (21.2%) consumed fruit four to six times weekly, while twenty-three (23.2%) consumed fruits daily. Thirty-five (35.3%) consumed two to three servings of fruits daily. Five (5%) consumed four to five fruits daily, while one (1%) consumed six or more fruits daily. According to a report from the Centers of Disease Control and Prevention (CDC), less than one third of Americans are eating enough fruits and vegetables. In addition, the same report stated, "a diet high in fruits and vegetables is associated with decreased risk for chronic disease" (CDC, 2005). The same findings were consistent with the diet history of the respondents.

The ingestion of dairy products was grouped together to include cheese, yogurt, cottage cheese, ice cream, margarine, butter, and soy-based dairy. Four (4%) of the respondents did not consume any dairy products on a weekly basis, with three (3%) of the respondents consuming one to three servings weekly. Twenty-three (23.7%) of respondents consumed dairy products four to six times weekly, while ten (10%) consumed dairy products daily. Forty (42%) consumed dairy products two to three times daily, while five (5%) consumed dairy products four to five times daily. Only two (2%) consumed more than six servings of dairy daily. According to the University of Illinois Extension, Americans were consuming more cream, sour cream, yogurt, and flavored milk in 2005 due to the increased availability of single serving sizes. Cheese was the number one (30 pounds per person) dairy product consumed, with milk coming in second. Of interest, individuals in Des Moines, Iowa consumed the most milk for a large city, at 18.7 gallons per person (University of Illinois Extension, 2005).

Bread and pasta were evaluated as a group. Foods included in this group were bread, cereal, white rice or pasta, brown rice, and whole grains. The number of servings in each group was scored as to how healthy the choices were. The maximum score was 20. A score of 15 to 20 was considered healthy, 10 to 14 considered moderately healthy, 5 to 9 healthy, and less than five unhealthy. Bread, pasta, and cereals are considered staple in most American diets. During a one-week period, 26 (26%) scored healthy, 52 (53%) scored moderately healthy, 13 (13%) scored fairly healthy and 8 (8 %) scored unhealthy. This score was based on the number of servings and the type of food. Three (3%) of the respondents stated they did not eat any foods from this group in a week.

The number of desserts or sweets eaten daily was important in the evaluation of adrenal stress/fatigue, as those individuals craved more simple carbohydrates or sweets in order to give them more energy. This creates unstable blood sugars with highs and lows. High insulin levels can be a factor in obesity because it is a fat storage hormone. Forty-five or 46% of respondents scored healthy on the question regarding sweets and dessert, with 52 or 54% scoring unhealthy. This broke down to nine (9%) never eating sweets and 3 (3%) eating desserts less than one per week. Thirty (30%) ate desserts one to three times per week, while ten (10%) ate desserts four to six times a week. Twenty-four (24.7%) ate desserts daily, while nineteen (19.5%) ate sweets two to three times daily. Two (2%) ate sweets four to five times daily.

The last question was the nutrition index which considered whether respondents were vegetarian or not. Four (4%) respondents stated they were vegetarian, with 93 (95%) being non-vegetarian. In summary, the nutrition guide was divided into four groups: very healthy (100-80), healthy (79-60), unhealthy (59-40) and very unhealthy (<39). None of the respondents scored very healthy, while thirty-four (34.3%) scored healthy. Sixty (60.6%) scored unhealthy and four (4%) scored very unhealthy.

The Lifestyle Guide

The lifestyle guide contained a number of questions regarding an exercise program, alcohol use, and supplement use. Dietary supplements refer to preparations designed to provide additional vitamins, minerals, essential fatty acids, or amino acids. Respondents taking supplements were interested in improving their health through use of supplements. Seventy-seven (77.3%) respondents took supplements while twenty-two (22.3%) stated they did not take any supplements.

Another important choice in the lifestyle guide was the question regarding smoking. Fourteen (14.4%) respondents smoked and 83 (85.6%) respondents did not smoke. Of the smokers, five were diagnosed with depression, three of the smokers had fibromyalgia and chronic fatigue, and three had hypothyroidism.

Sixty-six (68%) respondents had a regular exercise program of less than one hour daily. Thirty-one (31%) denied any exercise program and had a more sedentary lifestyle.

Along with exercise, the amount of sleep respondents received each night also had a bearing on their health. According to the National Institute of Health, 70 million Americans may be affected with chronic lack of sleep. This results in $15 billion in healthcare expenses and $50 billion in loss of productivity. Sixty-five (67%) respondents reported seven to eight hours of sleep, seven (7%) reported 9 or more hours of sleep and 25 (26%) reported six or less hours of sleep.

An additional area evaluated was whether or not respondents consumed alcoholic beverages. Seventy-three (75.2%) reported they did not consume any alcoholic beverages while twenty-four (24.8%) reported alcohol use.

The intake of water is important for a healthy body. Batmanghelidj (2000), suggests in his book that individuals should drink the amount of water equal to half their body weight in ounces, daily. (i.e. a 150 pound man should drink 75 ounces of water a day.) His research has found that dehydration can be a factor in many health problems including gastro-intestinal complaints, Alzheimer's disease, arthritis pain, migraine headaches, depression, fatigue, and hypertension. Thirty-one (31.9%) respondents drank less than 32 ounces of water daily, while 33 (34%) drank 24 to 32 ounces of water daily. Twenty-four (24.7%) drank 48 to 64 ounces of water daily, while only nine (9%) drank more than 64 ounces of water daily. The respondents' weight range was between 101 and 315 pounds, so the range of water intake should have been between 50 and 150 ounces of water daily. Since only 9 respondents stated they drank more than 64 ounces of water, it would seem that the majority of respondents were chronically dehydrated.

Sixty-eight (70.6) respondents carried some type of diagnosis while twenty-nine (29%) did not have any diagnosis. Many respondents carried more than one diagnosis, which is reflected in the data below:

Diagnosis		Taking Meds
Depression	35 (36%)	24.7%
Fibromyalgia	11 (11%)	6.5%
Sleep apnea	5 (5%)	0%
Anemia	3 (3%)	0%
Cardiovascular disease	5 (5%)	5%
Chronic fatigue	11 (11.3%)	0%
Hypothyroidism	25 (25.7%)	19%
Hypertension	23 (23.7%)	21%
Diabetes	8 (8%)	8%
Cancer	3 (3%)	3%

It has been this author's experience that those with fibromyalgia and chronic fatigue also had adrenal stress/fatigue. The diagnosis of GERD was not mentioned on the survey. However, 11 (11.3%) respondents took an acid stopping medication (H2 Blocker) which is a medication given for GERD. Kitchen (2001) describes several side effects of H2 Blockers, which include deficiency of intrinsic factor that is needed by the body to absorb vitamin B12. Other side effects may include malnutrition (acid is needed to absorb protein and minerals), toxicity, hypochlorhydria, parasites and degeneration of the gastric mucosa. Since digestion is so important in healing, correcting any digestion problems should be a high priority.

In summary, the lifestyle guide was divided into the following categories: very healthy lifestyle, healthy lifestyle, unhealthy lifestyle, and very unhealthy lifestyle. Eleven (11%) respondents scored very healthy and eleven (11%) scored healthy lifestyle. Seventy (70%) scored as having an unhealthy life style. This group of respondents participated in little or no exercise program, smoked and had at least one diagnosis. The final group of seven (7%) scored as having a very unhealthy lifestyle.

The Endocrine Guide

The Endocrine Guide involved a group of questions that indicated adrenal stress/fatigue. Group A addressed blood sugar handling while group B addressed liver/ gallbladder. Those with adrenal stress/fatigue tended to have more problems with low blood sugars and craved simple carbohydrates, sweets, coffee, or sodas. If the gallbladder is not functioning at an optimal rate or if the liver is toxic, these areas should be addressed in the healing process. As previously discussed, digestion (Group C) must be addressed for healing. Groups D and E were questions regarding thyroid function. The thyroid and adrenals work closely together, so individuals with adrenal stress/fatigue are often hypothyroid. In addition, they may have problems with autoimmune thryoiditis as noted when thyroid antibodies are elevated. Groups F and G were asked questions regarding the function of the pituitary gland. As symptoms of adrenal stress/fatigue increase, individuals may show increased stress on the pituitary gland, which indicates HPA axis dissociation. Questions H and I addressed symptoms of adrenal stress/fatigue. The final question (J) involved symptoms of B complex deficiency, because B vitamins are needed at the cellular level to assist in processing all fats, carbohydrates, and protein foods. B vitamins are also important in blood sugar handling and stress management. Therefore, higher scores indicated a chance of having adrenal stress/fatigue.

The aforementioned groups were divided into sections according to the total score. The first group (340-240) had a very high likelihood of adrenal stress/fatigue; the second group (239-169) had a high likelihood of adrenal stress/fatigue. The third group (168-99) had a medium likelihood of adrenal stress/fatigue, while the fourth group (98-40) had a low likelihood of adrenal stress/fatigue. The last group (<39) had a very low likelihood of adrenal stress/fatigue. One person (1%) had a very high likelihood of adrenal stress/fatigue while five (5%) had a high likelihood of adrenal stress/fatigue. Eighteen (18%) had a medium likelihood, while thirty-three had a low likelihood of adrenal stress/fatigue. Finally, forty-five had a very low likelihood of adrenal stress and fatigue.

Twenty-two of the respondents completed extra testing to rule out other causes of adrenal stress/fatigue. These included a hemoglobin test to rule out anemia and a blood sugar test to rule diabetes. Thyroid tests including thyroid-stimulating hormone (TSH), free T4, T3, and thyroid antibodies were completed to rule out hypothyroidism since this condition is often seen in individuals with adrenal stress/fatigue. Finally, an Adrenal Stress Index was completed. This test evaluated four cortisol levels throughout the day, as well as DHEA/cortisol level, 17 Hydroxyprogesterone, two insulin levels (one fasting and one post meal), salivary SIGA, and gliadin antibodies.

One hundred percent of the 21 respondents had normal hemoglobin and blood sugar levels, which ruled out anemia and diabetes as a cause of fatigue. One respondent had a TSH of 4.99, another had a TSH of 3.78, which may represent sub-clinical hypothyroidism. In addition, both of these respondents also had positive thyroid antibodies, which indicated autoimmune thryoiditis. The other respondents' TSH were within normal limits; however, four of these respondents also had positive thyroid antibodies.

Below is a chart with the summary of the findings of the 21 respondents. The first column represents the BMI of the respondents. Four of the respondents whose BMI scored obese had adrenal fatigue with low cortisol, two had adrenal stress, and four had both adrenal stress and fatigue. The next column represents the cortisol levels of each respondent. Adrenal fatigue refers to a low cortisol level, while adrenal stress refers to elevated cortisol level, and adrenal stress/fatigue represents cortisol which is both high and low throughout the day. Secretory IgA (SIgA) evaluates mucosal immunity by SIgA as a stress biomarker. SIgA are sensitive to increased cortisol/ DHEA ratio and sympathetic tone. DHEA measures DHEAs for the day the test was conducted and was recorded on how the body coped with stress. The body copes with stress in the following ways:

1. The body adapts to stress.
2. The body adapts to stress with a DHEA slump.
3. The body is in maladaption Phase I.
4. The body is in maladaption Phase II.
5. The body is in non-adaption with low reserves.
6. The body has high DHEA.
7. This phase is adrenal fatigue.

DHEA plays a role in cardiovascular disease, obesity, immune system, and lipid metabolism. The final column shows whether the respondent had a diagnosis, and if they had a diagnosis, whether they were taking medications for that diagnosis.

BMI	Free Corti-sol Rhythm	Survey	SIGA	DHEA	Diagnosis meds yes/no
23	fatigue	111	depressed	WNL	yes/yes
27.3	stress	177	depressed	borderline	yes/yes
46.3	stress	119	depressed	WNL	yes/no
42	fatigue	51	depressed	WNL	yes/yes
29	stress	NA	depressed	Phase I	yes/yes
28.2	stress	112	depressed	WNL	yes/yes
42	fatigue/stress	85	depressed	WNL	yes/yes
28.9	fatigue	27	depressed	Non-adapt	no
44.9	fatigue	160	borderline	WNL	yes /yes
19.6	fatigue	51	depressed	adrenal fatigue	no
43.8	fat/stress	79	depressed	phase II	yes/yes
25.2	fatigue	100	depressed	adrenal fatigue	yes/no
42.5	stress	110	depressed	phase I	yes/yes
27.3	fatigue	36	depressed	non-adapt	yes/yes
33.1	fatigue/stress	86	depressed	high DHEA	yes/no
26.6	stress	207	depressed	WNL	yes/yes
18.5	fatigue	174	depressed	adrenal fatigue	yes/yes
21.6	fatigue	112	depressed	non-adapt	yes/yes
20.7	fatigue/stress	81	depressed	WNL	no
19.8	fatigue/stress	193	borderline	WNL	yes/yes
45.4	fatigue/stress	335	depressed	WNL	yes/yes

It is interesting to note that the respondents' answers on the survey did not always correspond with the finding on the ASI. Therefore, when evaluating a client for adrenal stress/fatigue it is important to look at the whole picture (including medical, social and diet history) before recommending further testing as indicated.

CHAPTER 13

Conclusion, Implications and Recommendations

Conclusions and Implications

ADRENAL STRESS AND fatigue is just beginning to be recognized as a health issue for both sexes and for all ages. Currently Functional medicine professionals seem more aware of this issue than Western medicine professionals. It is now known that parents can pass down weakened adrenals to their offspring. Consequently, children are now experiencing adrenal stress/fatigue. In my practice, the youngest patient with adrenal fatigue has been age 5. This study has presented information on the importance of nutrition in relationship to health, especially adrenal stress/fatigue. Improvement in diet is vital whether practicing prevention or providing therapy for clients with adrenal stress/fatigue. As previously noted, correcting digestive disorders is an important first step in healing. H2 blockers should be discouraged and corrective therapies such as placing a client on digestive enzymes or a gluten free diet recommended. In the aforementioned section, four of the 21 respondents who completed the ASI were gluten-sensitive, while three of the 21 were borderline. To improve those respondents' digestion and health, recommending a gluten-free diet was important.

One of the study's results showed respondents were not eating healthy. In fact, many respondents did not realize how important a good diet was to health, even though there are increasingly more studies, lay literature, and media coverage, showing this. In 2002, the Health Organization completed a study in underdeveloped countries.

They noted that as economy improved, diets changed to include more high-energy foods, including more fats, sugars and fewer fruits and vegetables. Chronic disease that started in the womb and lasted throughout a lifetime was noted with poorer food choices. Hippocrates, the father of modern medicine, said well over 2000 years ago, "Let food be your medicine, and medicine be your food."

One limiting bias in the study related to the limited group living mainly in Iowa. However, there was no basis in relationship to income. All respondents were exposed to media discussing the importance of improved nutrition. Expanding the study to include individuals in other states, as well as city and rural areas, would provide more diversity to the study.

The responses to questions in the Nutrition Guide, Lifestyle Guide, and the BMI rate some of those surveyed in higher risk groups for developing adrenal stress/fatigue. High risk responses correlate to poorer choices of food and the lack of fruits and vegetables. This was noted on a number of surveys as shown in the increased use of caffeinated beverages and the excessive intake of sweets and simple carbohydrates.

The Endocrine Guide brought to light the facts that are often seen in individuals with adrenal stress/fatigue. These included B-Complex deficiency, blood sugar handling (often related to blood sugars following an up and down pattern), digestion issues, and liver gallbladder toxicity. Many individuals with chronic stress also had problems with hormone regulation such as estrogen dominance.

Recommendation for Further Research

This author recommends that further research be conducted on this subject involving a larger study being conducted on all age groups. This would assist in improved statistical analysis with more advanced methods. At the same time, confusing questions could be tailored to provide more detail. It would be interesting to repeat this survey after improvement in nutrition and other recommended therapy was implemented to look at the extent of healing. One method of looking at the extent of healing would include the use of the Adrenal Stress Index (ASI), both as screening and post therapy if symptoms of adrenal stress and fatigue were present. It is recommended that both the Nutrition Guide and Lifestyle Guide be improved with questions related to daily use rather than weekly, because this made the statistical analysis more difficult.

Such a study would have many variables. This could be a disadvantage because each individual could require a different approach regarding supplement use, etc. The nutritional recommendations could be standardized with the same guidelines given to each respondent.

Summary

This study was divided into two sections. The first section discussed adrenal stress/fatigue, incidence of, signs and symptoms, and a variety of therapies that include nutritional, herbal and lifestyle changes. A comparison was completed between Western medicine and Functional medicine regarding the identification of and therapies for adrenal stress/fatigue. This was accomplished by means of a literature search.

The second section consisted of a survey of clients who visited the Natural Health Center in Atlantic, Iowa, as well as from an e-mail listing. The goal was to identify the number of respondents completing the survey who had the likelihood of adrenal stress/fatigue. The survey looked at nutrition, lifestyle, and endocrine function of each respondent.

CHAPTER 14

Protocols

Protocols

Maintenance supplements:

Catalyn®: 1-2 tabs, 3 times daily; whole food multiple vitamin.
Juice Plus+®: 2 capsules, 2 times daily; whole food fruit and vegetable capsules.

Adrenal Support: Primary

Drenamine®: 2-3 tabs 3 times daily; contains Cataplex® G (B-Complex), Cataplex® C, and Drenatrophin® to rebuild adrenals. May be used long term.
Cataplex® B: 2 tabs, 3 times daily (contains additional B vitamins).
Trace Minerals B12TM: 1tab three times daily

Adrenal Support: Additional choices:

AdrenalTM *Desiccated*: 1-2 tabs 3 times daily. To be used short term 1-2 months. Helps with immediate energy but will not help adrenal glands repair.

Drenatrophin PMG®: 2 tabs 3 times daily. Contains no gluten as Drenamine®

Cataplex® C: 2 tabs 3 times daily, if not taking Drenamine®. (Note: 15 mg of whole food Vitamin C equals 1500 mg of ascorbic acid)

HPA Axis support:

Symplex® F: (female) support ovaries, adrenal, thyroid, and pituitary. 1 tab, 3 times daily for 4 months.

Symplex® M: (male) support testes, adrenal, thyroid, and pituitary. 1 tab, 3 times daily for 4 months.

Paraplex®: supports thyroid, pituitary, adrenal, and pancreas. 1 tab 3 times Daily for 4 months.

Digestive Support:

Gastrex®: 1 to 2, 3 times daily 15 minutes before meals

AF Betafood®: 2, 3 times daily

Multizyme®: 1 to 2 with meals or

Enzycore: 1 to 2 with meals or

Zypan®: 1 to 2 with meals, contains HCL

Herbal Support

Gymnema: 1 tab, 2 times daily for carb craving and lower blood sugar.

Rhodiola and Ginseng Complex (Panex Ginseng): 1 tab 2-4 times daily. Both stimulate adaptogens.

Tribulus: 1 tab 1-3 times daily. Benefit growth hormone regulation via HP axis; increases testosterone in men.

Licorice: High Grade 2.5 ml diluted water daily. Caution if hypertension.

Adrenal Complex 1-3 tabs daily. Combination of Rehmannia and licorice.

Rehmannia: Liquid 5 ml 1-3 daily. No concern regarding blood pressure.

Ashwaganda: 5 ml daily. Use for patients on prednisone to support adrenals. helps cope with stress. Use in high or low cortisol levels.

Eleuthero: 5 ml daily. Adaptogen.

Liquid herbal combinations. (Note: These dosages reflect herbs from MediHerb)

Tonic formula for Phase 2 Adrenal Stress:
   Rehmannia 1:1: 30 ml (adrenal support).
   Echinacea Premium 1:2: 20 ml (immune support).
   Valerian 1:2: 20 ml calming.
   Ashwaganda 1:2: 30 ml. Mix together dosage 8 ml 2 times daily.

Tonic formula for Phase 3 Adrenal Stress
   Licorice 1:1: 15 ml may substitute Rehmannia if blood pressure concerns.
   Astragalus 1:2: 25 ml tonic and adaptogen.
   Ginkgo 2:1: 20 ml antioxidant and promote mental clarity.
   St John's Wort 1:2: 20 ml support emotional and mental health.
   Eleuthero 1:2: 20 ml. Mix together. Dosage is 8 ml, 2 times daily.

Phosophatidylserine
PS is a phospholipid found in cell membranes such as brain cells.
   Dosage varies with different products from 880 mg to 3000 mg daily.
   Use 1 to 2 hours before high cortisol levels to normalize cortisol. Especially helpful for sleep when nighttime cortisol is elevated.

RESOURCES

Complementary Care Center: LLC: 712 243-2800, or www.compcarehealth.com

Natural Health Center: 712 243-2800, or www.nahealthctr.com Kerry Sauser ARNP, ND, PhD practices integrative functional healthcare

Standard Process and MediHerb: 800 558-8740, or www.standardprocess.com Whole food supplements and herbal products

NSA, LLC: www.juiceplus.com Whole food supplements of fruit and vegetable blends Juice Plus+® products

Bezwecken: 800 743-2256, Women's Health Care Products including sublingual Bio-identical hormones, vaginal creams, and suppositories

Nordic Naturals: 800 662-2544 ext 17 or www.nordicnaturals.com pure, fresh fish oils

Analytic Research Labs (ARL): 800 528-4067, Hair Testing Lab

DiagnosTechs: 800 878-3787, www.diagnostechs.com, hormone both male and female, Adrenal, and digestive saliva kits

Radiant Heal Imaging: 1 866-240-9659 www.radianthealthimaging. com Thermography of breasts or total body

Genova Diagnostics: 800 522-4762 www.genvodiagnostics.com nutritional Gastrointestinal, immune, and endocrine testing

Great Plains Laboratory: 800288-0383 www.greatplainslaboratory.com nutritional Testing, specializes in testing for those with mental health issues, children

Metametrix Clinical Lab: 800 221-4640 www.metametrix.com

Trace Elements, INC.: 972-250-6410 www.labinc.com hair testing lab

BioHealth Diagnostics: 800-570-2000 www.biodia.com saliva testing, hormone, adrenalStool testing

APPENDIX

APPENDIX A:

Survey with scoring

THE SURVEY BELOW is part of my dissertation for my Doctor of Philosophy in Holistic Nutrition from Clayton College of Natural Health. The subject of my dissertation is adrenal stress/fatigue. This survey will assist me in gathering information to determine if adrenal fatigue is a likely missed diagnosis. This survey will ask a variety of questions regarding your diet, lifestyle, medical history, and medication and supplement use. Since some of this information may be considered personal, all the information will be kept private. Those who have the right to look at this study records are those completing the study and the Clayton College IRB committee. Although records can be opened by court order, they will be kept confidential to the extent of the law. Please answer all questions truthfully. Thank you for your time.

General Information:
1.   What is your height? _____ (convert to inches)
     Weight? _____

     To be used to determine BMI

2.   How old are you? _____

3.   What is your sex? Male_____Fe_____

4.   What is your nationality?

     _____African American

     _____Hispanic or Latino

_____Caucasian

_____Asian, Asian American

_____Other

5. What state and town do you live in? _____

Diet and Nutrition Questions:

Please refer to the last six months when answering these questions.

1. How many times do you eat out weekly? Please include fast food or take out. _____ *Max is 5; Healthy is 4*

    None=5   If fast food
    1-3 =4   None= 1
    4-6 = 2   1-10= 0
    7-10 = 1
    >10 = 0

2. What types of beverages do you drink on an average day? Please state how many cups or 8 ounce glasses.

    _____

    Combine questions 2 and 6

    Max score is 5 Healthy = 4 If respondent has score of 5, 1 point deducted for regular coffee, or soft drink

Regular coffee	1
Decaffeinated coffee	0
Regular black tea	1
Regular green tea	1
Regular herbal tea	1
Decaffeinated tea	1
Regular soft drink	1
Diet soft drink	1
Water	5
Milk whole	0
2% & 1%, skim milk	0
Soy milk	0
Almond milk	1

3   How many servings of breads, pasta, cereals, or grains do you eat each week? Please state if they are whole grain or white.

_____

	Never,	1/ wk	-3/ wk	4-6/ wk	daily	2-3/day	4-5/day	> 6 daily
Bread	5	4	3	2	0	0	0	0
Cereal	0	1	3	4	5	3	0	0
White rice	5	4	2	1	0	0	0	0
Brown rice & Whole grains	0	1	3	4	5	4	1	0

4.   How many servings of vegetables do you eat weekly?

_____

Question 14 and 15 combined Max score is 25, Healthy = 15

Fruits & vegetables	Never	<1/wk	1-3/wk	4-6/wk	Daily	2-3/day	4-5/day	>6/day
Servings of vegetables	0	1	2	3	4	5	5	5
Salad	0	1	2	3	5	5	—	—
Potato	5	4	2	1	0	0	—	—
French fries	5	3	1	0	0	0	—	—
Serving of fruit	0	1	2	3	4	5	5	—

5.   How many fruits do you eat weekly?

_____

6.   How many servings of milk or dairy products do eat weekly?

_____

Max score for dairy is 27, healthy=20

Dairy	Never	<1/wk	1-3/wk	4-6/wk	Daily	2-3/day	4-5/day	>6/day
Cheese	5	4	3	2	1	0	0	—
Yogurt cottage cheese	0	1	3	4	5	4	—	—
Ice cream	5	4	2	0	0	0	—	—
Margarine	5	4	1	0	0	0	0	—
Butter	3	4	4	3	3	0	0	—
Soy based dairy	0	2	3	2	2	0	—	—

7. How many sweets or desserts do you eat weekly?_____

Max score for sweets and snacks is 15, healthy =12

Sweets and Snacks	Never	<1/wk	1-3/wk	4-6/wk	Daily	2-3/day	4-5/day	>6/day
Sweet roll, doughnut,	5	4	2	0	0	0	0	0
Candy	5	4	1	0	0	0	0	0
Pie, cake	5		4	2	1	0	0	0

8. Are you a vegetarian? Yes   No

   Yes——vegetarian   5
   Yes —-vegan   2
   No—-   0

9. Do you take any supplements, vitamins, herbs or homeopathy remedies? _____

   Yes 2
   No 0

10. If you answered yes to question 9, please list all supplements you take on a regular basis, including the brand name of each.

_____

_____

Lifestyle Questions:

1. On an average how much sleep do you get each night?

_____

2. On an average day, what time do you go to bed?

_____

3. On an average day, what time do you get up?

_____

Combine questions 1, 2, and 3
Max 4 Healthy 3 8-9 hours = 4, 6-7 = 3, 5-6= 2, < 5= 0

4. Do you exercise weekly? Yes No How many times a week? _____

5. What type of exercise do you enjoy?

_____

Question 4 and 5 combined
Do not exercise   0
1-2 hours per day   3
3-4 hours per day   1
> 4 hours day   0

6. Do you smoke or use some form of tobacco? Yes = 0 No = 5

7. Do you drink any alcoholic beverages, if so how many ounces weekly?

(1 drink is 12 ounce of beer, 4 ounces of wine or one shot of hard liquor.)

_____

No drinks   5
1 drink   3

2 drinks   1

Greater than 2 drinks = 0

8.   How many ounces of water do you drink daily?

_____

9.   Please circle any health issues diagnosed with.

Diabetes   Hypertension   Fibromyalgia   Sleep apnea

Anemia   Cardiovascular disease   Depression

Chronic fatigue   Thyroid disease

Condition	Diagnosed with	Taking medications for
Cardiovascular disease	Yes = 1 No = 0	Yes =1 No = 0
Depression	Yes = 1 No= 0	Yes = 1 No = 0
Diabetes	Yes = 1 No = 0	Yes =1 No = 0
Hypertension	Yes =1 No = 0	Yes = 1 No = 0
Thyroid Disease	Yes = 1 No = 0	Yes = 1 No = 0
Anemia	Yes = 1 No = 0	Yes = 1 No = 0
Sleep apnea	Yes = 1 No = 0	Yes = 1 No = 0
Fibromyalgia	Yes = 1 No = 0	Yes = 1 No = 0
Chronic fatigue	Yes = 1 No = 0	Yes = 1 No = 0

10.   Please list all prescription medications you are taking and indicate their purpose.

_____

Please rate each item below by the following scale. If an item does not apply to you leave blank. Remember you are considering only the last six months.

A = mild (once or twice a month):

B = moderate (several times per month):

C = severe (daily)

Group A: Blood sugar handling

_____Eat when nervous   _____Excessive appetite

_____Hungry between meals _____Irritable before meals

_____Gets shaky if hungry   _____Afternoon headache

_____Fatigue relieved by eating

_____Lightheaded if meals delayed

_____Overeating sweets upsets

_____Crave candy, soda or coffee in afternoons

_____Awaken after few hours sleep, difficulty getting back to sleep

_____Moods of depression

_____Abnormal craving for sweets

Blank = 0 A = 1 B = 2 C = 3

Higher the score increased problems with low blood sugar

Group B: Liver/Gallbladder

_____Dizziness   _____Worrier, feels insecure

_____Feeling queasy; headache   _____Dry skin

_____Greasy foods upsets   _____Light colored stools

_____Burning feet   _____Skin peels soles of feet

_____Pain between shoulder blades   _____Blurred vision

_____Laxative use   _____Stools alternate from soft to watery

_____Itching skin, feet   _____History of gallbladder attacks

_____Sneezing attacks   _____Excessive hair falling out

_____Bad breath   _____Intolerance of dairy foods

_____Bitter, metallic taste in mouth in AM

_____Burning or itching rectum

_____Difficult or painful BM's

_____Crave sweets

Higher the score needs Gall bladder cleanse and estrogen dominance

Group C: Digestion

_____Loss of taste for meat

_____Lower bowel gas several hours after eating

_____Eating relieves burning stomach

_____Coated tongue

_____Pass large amounts of foul-smelling gas

_____Irritable bowel

_____Indigestion 30 min. to 4 hours after meals

_____Gas shortly after eating

_____Stomach bloating after eating

Blank = 0   A = 1   B = 2   C = 3

Higher score increased problems with digestion

Group D: Hyperactive thyroid (associated with adrenal stress)

_____Insomnia   _____Nervousness

_____Can't gain weight   _____Intolerance to heat

_____Highly emotional   _____Flushes easily

_____Night sweats   _____Heart palpitates

_____Thin, moist skin   _____Inward trembling

_____Pulse fast at rest

_____Increased appetite no weight gain

_____Eyelids & face twitch

_____Irritable & restless

_____Can't work under pressure

Blank = 0   A = 1   B = 2   C = 3

Higher score increased problems hyperactive thyroid

Group E: Hypoactive thyroid

_____Weight increased   _____Decreased appetite

_____Easily fatigue   _____Ringing in ears

_____Sleepy during day   _____Sensitive to cold

_____Dry or scaly skin   _____Constipation

_____Mental sluggishness   _____Hair course falls out

_____Headaches on arising, subsides during day

_____Slow pulse below 65   _____Urinate frequently

_____Impaired hearing   _____Reduced Initiative

Blank = 0   A = 1   B = 2   C = 3

Higher score increased problems hypoactive thyroid and adrenal fatigue

Group F: Hyperactive pituitary

_____Failing Memory   _____Low blood pressure

_____Sex drive increased   _____Splitting headaches

_____Decreased sugar tolerance

Blank = 0   A = 1   B = 2   C = 3

Higher score increased problems hyperactive pituitary increased adrenal stress

Group G: Hypoactive pituitary

_____Abnormal thirst   _____Bloating of abdomen

_____Weight gain around waist   _____Sex drive reduced

_____Tendency to ulcers, colitis   _____Menstrual disorders

_____Increased sugar tolerance

_____Young girls: lack of menstrual periods

Blank = 0   A = 1   B = 2   C = 3

Higher score increased problems hypoactive pituitary and HPA axis disregulation

Group H: Adrenal stress

_____Dizziness _____Headaches _____Hot flashes

_____Increased blood pressure

_____Hair growth on face (female) _____Restless legs

_____Loss of weight without reason

_____Masculine tendencies (female)

_____Nervous under pressure _____Increasing PMS

_____Do best work late at night

_____like to sleep late in AM

Group I: Adrenal fatigue

_____Weakness, dizziness

_____Chronic fatigue not relieved by rest

_____Low blood pressure _____Nails, weak, have ridges

_____endency to hives _____Arthritic tendencies

_____Increased Perspiration _____Bowel disorders

_____Poor circulation _____Swollen ankles

_____Crave salt _____Brown spots or bronzing of skin

_____Increased allergies _____Weakness after colds

_____Get a second burst of energy after 9 PM

_____Exhaustion _____Don't feel well

_____Decreased tolerance to cold

_____Get best rest between 7 & 9 AM

_____Respiration disorders

Blank = 0   A = 1   B = 2   C = 3

Higher score increased problems adrenal fatigue

Group J: B-Complex deficiency.

Needed to assist in processing fats, carbohydrates, and protein and stress handling

_____Apprehension _____Irritability _____

_____Morbid fears _____Forgetfulness

_____Never seems well _____Indigestion

_____Poor appetite _____Craving sweets

_____Muscular soreness _____Depression

_____Noise sensitivity _____Acoustic hallucinations

_____Weakness _____Tendency to cry without reason

_____Hair coarse, thinning _____Fatigue

_____Skin sensitive to touch _____Nervousness

_____Headache _____Insomnia _____Anxiety

_____Anorexia _____Inability to concentrate

_____Frequent stuffy nose, infections

_____Allergy to some foods _____Loose joints

Blank = 0   A = 1   B = 2   C = 3

The higher score increases the likelihood of adrenal fatigue (Rosen 2007).

APPENDIX B

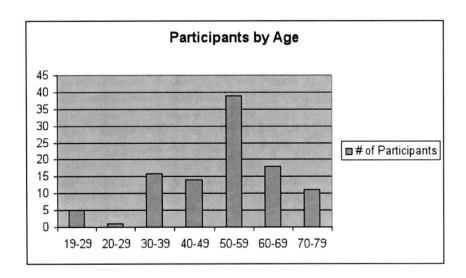

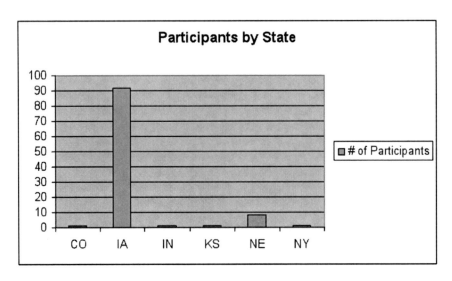

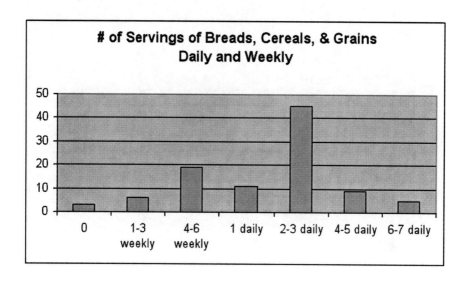

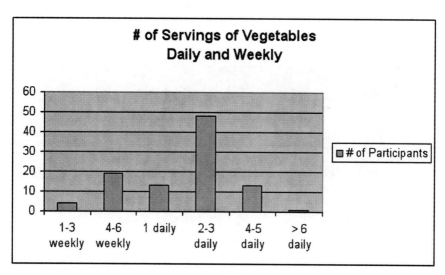

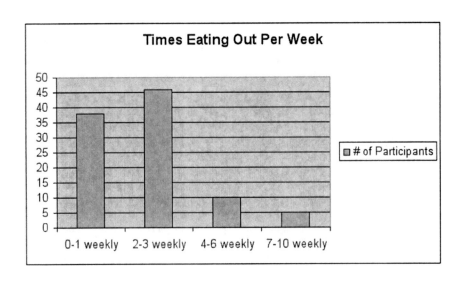

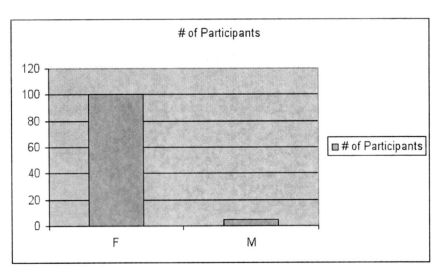

APPENDIX C

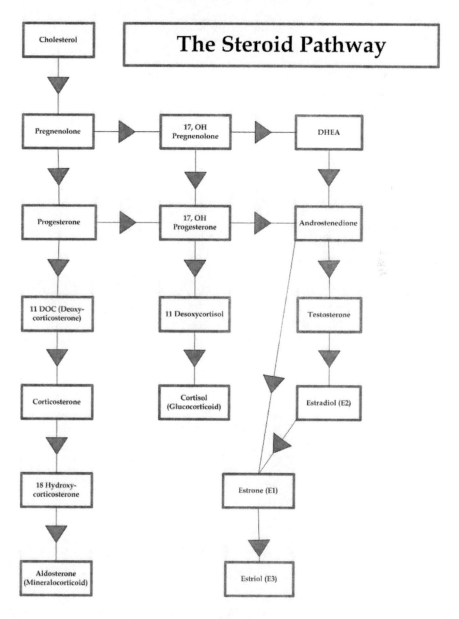

The Steroid Pathway

Cholesterol → Pregnenolone → 17, OH Pregnenolone → DHEA

Pregnenolone → Progesterone

17, OH Pregnenolone → 17, OH Progesterone

DHEA → Androstenedione

Progesterone → 11 DOC (Deoxy-corticosterone)

17, OH Progesterone → 11 Desoxycortisol

Androstenedione → Testosterone

11 DOC (Deoxy-corticosterone) → Corticosterone

11 Desoxycortisol → Cortisol (Glucocorticoid)

Testosterone → Estradiol (E2)

Corticosterone → 18 Hydroxy-corticosterone

Estradiol (E2) → Estrone (E1)

18 Hydroxy-corticosterone → Aldosterone (Mineralocorticoid)

Estrone (E1) → Estriol (E3)

DEFINITION OF TERMS

Adrenocorticotropic: (ACTH) A pituitary hormone that stimulates the adrenal cortex to produce steroid hormones.

Aldosterone: Steroid hormone secreted by the adrenal cortex, that controls mineral and water balance.

Alternative medicine: An outdated term that refers to everything outside the realm of conventional medicine. It is outdated since alternative medicine is now mainstream medicine.

Anabatic: The process of building up.

Corticotrophin Releasing Hormone: Polypeptide hormone and neurotransmitter involved in stress response.

Catabolism: A set of pathways that break down molecules into smaller units to release energy. It provides the chemical energy necessary for maintenance and growth of cells.

Complementary medicine: Combines conventional therapies with alternative therapies. Promoters of "complementary medicine" often prescribed drugs and surgery but use this phrase to avoid appearing totally out of touch with health trends.

Conventional medicine: Refers to the traditional medical training offered through mainstream medical schools. This is a drug and surgery approach to medicine that largely excludes nutrition, wellness, mind body medicine, patient education and other natural therapies.

Dehydroepiandrosterone: (DHEA) A steroid hormone synthesized from cholesterol and secreted by the adrenal glands

Diabetes: A disease in which the pancreas produces insufficient amounts of insulin or in which cells fail to respond to insulin as in insulin resistance.

Eastern medicine: Looks at whole patient, the whole body, the whole experience, and never believes that just treating one organ or using one chemical, drug, or herb is the answer to any health condition.

Estrogen: Steroid hormone, produced mainly by ovaries: stimulates development of female secondary sexual characteristics.

HPA axis: Hypothalamus, pituitary and adrenals

Hyperpituitarism: Excessively high activity of the pituitary gland.

Hypoglycemia: Low blood sugar

Hypopituitarism: Failure of pituitary gland to produce hormones.

Integrative / Functional medicine: A recent term that that describes a more balanced, welcome approach to using natural therapies alongside conventional therapies. Integrative medicine is now taught in 28 major medical schools, but is not practiced by many health care providers. Functional medicine uses evidence based, proven methods in health care.

Organized medicine: A collection of organizations that promote conventional medicine such as the FDA, and American Medical Association.

Secretory IGA: Main immunoglobulin found in mucous secretions including tears, saliva, colostrum, intestinal and vaginal fluids. It provides protection against microbes that multiply in body secretion.

Pernicious anemia: A severe form of anemia found mostly in senior citizens, that results from the body's inability to absorb Vitamin B12. Symptoms include weakness, breathing difficulties, and weight loss.

Pregnenolone: Steroid hormone synthesized from cholesterol.

Progesterone: Sex hormone produced by women, first by the corpus luteum of the ovary then later by the placenta to maintain pregnancy

Protomorphogen (PMG): Extracts which contain "cell determinates" from specific organs and glands for clinical use.

Testosterone – Male steroid hormone produced in the testicles which is responsible for secondary sex characteristics in males.

Thyroiditis: Inflammation of thyroid.

Traditional Chinese or TCM: Involves treatment of patients using the fundamental approaches of healing developed over the last 4000 years in China. These may include acupuncture and Chinese herbs.

Western medicine: Refers to the type of medicine practiced in the West primarily the United States and Western Europe.

REFERENCES

Aardal, E., Holm, A.C. (1995) Cortisol in saliva-reference ranges and relation to cortisol in serum. *European Journal of Clinical Chemistry and Clinical Biochemistry* December; 33(12):927-32. Abstract retrieved June 13, 2009 from PubMed database

Adams, M., (2006). Systems of medicine explained: conventional, alternative complementary and more *News Target*, 5. Retrieved May 5, 2006 from http://www.newstarget.com/019365.html

Adrenal fatigue syndrome (2006). Retrieved May 26, 2006 from http://www.jigsawhealth.com/article_print.aspx?articleID=38.

Adrenal fatigue: what causes it? (2007) Retrieved September 12, 2007 from http://www.mayoclinic.com/health/adrenal-fatigue/ANO1583.

Adrenal gland disorders (2003). *Merck Manual* Retrieved June 4, 2006 from http://www.merke.com/mmhe/print/sec13ch164ch164a.html

Adrenal fatigue: what causes it? (2007) Retrieved September 12, 2007 from http://www.mayoclinic.com/print/adrenal-fatigue/ANO1583? METHOD=print

Ahrens, T., Deuschie, M. Krumm, B., vander Pompe, G., den Boer, J ., Lederbogen, F., (2008). Pituitary-adrenal and sympathetic nervous system responses to stress in women remitted from recurrent major depression, *Psychosomatic Medicine,* May; (7094):461-7, E pub 2008 Mar 31. Abstract retrieved June 13, 2009 from PubMed Database

Albert-Matesz, R., (2005). Beat your sugar cravings. *Mother Earth News* (2010), 81- 84.

Alderling, M., (2006). The demand control model and circadian saliva variations in a swedish population based sample [Electronic Version]. *Biomed Central*, 1471-2458. Retrieved March 3, 2008.

Alleger, I.(2001). *Balancing hormones and breast cancer.* Retrieved December 12, 2007

Amick, B., McDonough, P., Chang, H., Rogers, W., Piepers, W., Duncan, G., (2002). Relationship between all-cause mortality and cumulative working life course psychosocial and physical exposures in the united states labor market from 1968 to 1992. *Psychosmatic Medicine 64, 370-381.* Retrieved March 9, 2008 from http://www.psychosomaticmedicine.org/cgi/content/abstract/64/3/370?maxtoshow=&HITS

Anderson. D., (2008). Assessment and nutraceutical management of stress-induced adrenal dysfunction. *Integrative medicine: a clinician's journal* Oct/Nov Vol. 7 No. 5 p.18-25

Arlt, W., Allolio, B., (2003). Adrenal insufficiency. *Lancet,* 361 (9372), 1881. Retrieved October 16, 2007 from http://web.ebscohost.com/ehost/delivery?vid=9&hid=116&sid=62c06ac0-e7da-4d62-9cb

Association American Medical Colleges. School Curriculum: AAMC. Retrieved June 6, 2006 from http://services.aamc.org/currdir/section2/courses.cfm

Association American Medical Colleges: Tomorrow's Doctors (2006). *Curriculum Directory.* Retrieved March 29/2006 from http://service.aamc.org/currdir/sction2/courses.cfm

Barker, J., (2005). The naturopathic approach to adrenal dysfunction. *Townsend Letter for Doctors and Patients.* Retrieved March 3, 2008, http://findarticles.com/p/articles/mi_mOISW/is-259-260/ai_n12417485/print

Barston, S., Toscano, M., (2008). *Healthy eating tips for a healthy diet.* Retrieved July 18, 2008 from http://helpguide.veg/life/healthy_eating_diet.html

Baschetti, R., (2003). Organic vs. cultural explanations of chronic fatigue syndrome and fibromyalgia. *Journal of the America Medical Association,* 289(11), 1385-.

Baschetti, R., Chester, A. C., Devitt, N. F., & Komaroff, A. L., (1998). Chronic fatigue syndrome. *Journal of the America Medical Association,* 279(6), 431-433.

Baschetti, R., Teitelbaum, J. E., Bird, B., Weiss, A., Gould, L., Friedman, T. C., et al. (1999). Low-dose hydrocortisone for chronic fatigue syndrome. *Journal of the America Medical Association,* 281(20), 1887-1889.

Batmanghelidj, F., (2000). *Your body's cries for water.* Global Health Solutions, Inc., Falls City

Be healthier: eat red, orange, and green food. (2006) Retrieved June 28/2006 from http://www.msnbc.msn.com/id/13546647/from/ET/print/1/displaymode/1098/

Bee, P. (2004). Complementary aid. *Times, the United Kingdom.* Retrieved October 16, 2007 from http//www.web.ebscohost.com/ehost/detail?vid=7&hid+116&sid=62c)6ac)-e7da4da-4d62-9cb2-1

Bellingrath, S.,Weigl, T., Kudielka, B.(2008). Cortisol disregulation in school teachers in relation to burnout, vital exhaustion, and effort-reward-imbalance. *Biology Psychology.* Retrieved March 9, 2008, from PubMed database

Bharat Sangani, D., (2005). Ask the doctor: more tips to help relieve your stress. *Sun Herald.* Biloxi, MS.

Bierhaus, A., (2003). *A mechanism converting psychosocial stress into mononuclear cell activation.* Retrieved March 09, 2008

Blacker, C. V. R., Greenwood, D. T., Wesnes, K. A., Wilson, R., Wood-ward, C., Howe, I., et al. (2004). Effect of galantamine hydrobromide in chronic fatigue syndrome: a randomized controlled trial. *Journal of the America Medical Association,* 292(10), 1195-1204.

Bone, K., (no date given) Chronic fatigue syndrome and its herbal treatment. *MediHerb Clinical*

Bone, K., (1989). Licorice—the universal herb part one. *MediHerb Professional Review.* 10 (4) 1-3.

Bone, K., (1996). *Clinical applications of ayurvedic and chinese herbs.* Warwick: Phytotherapy Press.

Bone, K., (2001). *Clinical applications of ayurvedic and chinese herbs.* Queenlands: Phytotherapy Press

Bone, K., (2003). *A Clinical guide to blending liquid herbs.* China: Churchill Livingston

Bone, K., (2005) Herbs with tonic, adaptogenic, adrenal tonic, and nervine activity. *MediHerb Professional Review* 58 *(10)*1-2

Bone, K., (2007). *MediHerb product catalog.* (pp. 10-27): MediHerb.

Bone, K., Mills, S. (2000). *Principles and practices of phytotherapy.* London: Churchill Livingstone

Bone, K., Morgan, M. (2001). Gymnema sylvestre-gymnema. *MediHerb Professional Review.* Retrieved October 13, 2007, Number 75

Bone, K., Morgan, M., (2005) Licorice—the universal herb part 2. *MediHerb professional review.* June 1, p. 1-4

Bowen, R. A., (1998). *Adrenal medullary hormones.* Retrieved June 4, 2006 from http:www.vivo.colostate.edu/hbooks/pathphys/endocrine/adrenal/gluco.html

Bowen, R. A., (1999). *Mineralcorticoids* . Retrieved June 4, 2006 from http://www.vivocolostate.edu/hbooks/pathphys/endocrine/adrenal/mineralo.html

Bowen, R. A., (2001a). *Adrenal steroids.* Retrieved June 4, 2006 from http://www.vivocolostate.edu/hbooks/pathphys/endocrine/adrenal/steroids.html

Bowen, R. A., (2001b) *Steroidogeneisis.* Retrieved June 4, 2006 from http://www.vivo.colostate.edu/hbooks/pathphys/endocrine//basics/steroidogensis.html

Bowen, R. A, (2002). *Functional anatomy of the adrenal gland.* Retrieved June 4, 2006 from http:www.vivo.colostate.edu/hbooks/path phys/endocrine/adrenal/anatomy.html.

Bowen, R., (2006). Glucocorticoids: *colorado state.* Retrieved June 4, 2006 from http://www.vivo.colostate.edu/hbooks/pathphys/endocrine/adrenal/gluco.html

Brooke, A., Monson, J., (2005). Addison's disease. *Medicine, 33,* (11), 20-22. Abstract retrieved March 10, 2008 from http://www.science direct.com/science?_ob=ArticleURL&-udi=B82YB-4KY9TRY-9&_us

Brown, G., (2000). Effects of anabolic precursors on serum testosterone concentrations and adaptations to resistance training in young men. *International Journal of Sport Nutrition and Exercise Metabolism,* 10(3), 340-359. Abstract retrieved April 6, 2008 from http://www.ncbinlm.nih.gov/pubmed/10997957

Carpenter, L., (2004). Cerebrospinal fluid corticotropin-releasing factor and perceived early-life stress in depressed patients and healthy control subjects *Neuropsychopharmacology* 777-784. [Electronic Version]. Retrieved March 3, 2008.

Center of Disease Control. (2002). *Diet, nutrition and the prevention of chronic disease: report of a joint WHO/FAO expert consultation.* Retrieved July 11, 2009 from http://www.eldis.org/go/topic/resource-giudes/health/nutrition-anddisease&id=

Center of Disease Control. (2003). *Behavioral risk factor surveillance system survey data* [Electronic Version]. Retrieved March 16, 2008.

Center of Disease Control (2006). *CFS possible causes.* Retrieved October 18, 2007 from   http://www.cdc.gov/print.do?url=http:www.cdc.gov/cfs/cfs/cfscauses.htm

Center of Disease Control. (2007). *Fruit and vegetable consumption among adults*—United States, 2005]. Retrieved March 16, 2008 from
http:www.cdc.gov/mmwr/preview/mmwrhtml/mm5610a2.htm.

Chaudhuri, A., & Behan, P. O., (2004). Fatigue in neurological disorders. *Lancet,* 363(9413), 978-988.

Children's Hospital of Wisconsin (2006). *Disorders affecting the adrenal glands.* Retrieved June 4, 2006 from http://www.chw.org/display/PPF/DocID/22683/router.asp

Cicero, A. (2004). Effects of Siberian ginseng on elderly quality of life: a randomized trail. Arch Gerontol Geriatr Suppll, 9, 69-73. Abstract retrieved April 1, 2008 from http://www.ncbi.nlm.nih.gov/pubmed/15207399?ordinal-pos=4&itool=EntrezSystem 2.PEntr

Clinical Research. *Adrenal stress index salivary testing.* Kent Diagnos-Techs, INC.

Cohen, M., Sandler, L., Hrbek, A., Davis, R., Eisenberg, D., Polices pertaining to complementary and alternative medical therapies in a random sample of 39 academic health centers. *Alternative therapies,* Jan/Feb, 2005, 36-40

Cohen, (1991). Psychological stress and susceptibility to common cold [Electronic Version]. *New England Journal of Medicine* 606-612. Retrieved March 9, 2008.

Coleman, C., Herbert, J., Reddy, P., (2003). The effects of panax ginseng on quality of life. *Journal of Clinical Pharmacy and Therapeutics.* Feb:28(1)5-15. Abstract retrieved April 7, 2008 from PubMed data base

Cowman, T. M. D., (2007). Diseases of adrenal cortex insufficiency—asthma, allergies, eczema. *In The Four Fold Path to Healing,* 179-195.

Craeford, A., (1997). *Herbal remedies for women.* Roseville: Prima Publishing

Devanur, L., Kerr, J., (2006). Chronic fatigue syndrome. *Journal of Clinical Virology, 37* (3), 139-150 Retrieved March 10, 2008 from http://www.sciencedirect.com/science?_ob=articleURL&_udi=B6VJV-4KWTFPT- 2&_us

Donaldson, R., (2006). Rhodiola rosea. *Insight Journal.* Retrieved January 30, 2011 from http//www.anxiety-and-depression-solutions.com/printer/Rhodiola_rosea_printer.php

Disorders affecting the adrenal glands [Electronic Version]. Retrieved June 4, 2006.

Drasch, G., Roider, G., (2002). Assessment of hair mineral analysis commercially offered in Germany. *Journal of Trace Elements in Medicine and Biology,* 16, 27-31. Abstract retrieved March 23, 2008 from http://www.sciencedirect.com/science?_ob=articleURL&_udi=B7GJC-4GWPPS5-5&_us

Dr Royal Lee, DDS, (2001-2003). Retrieved January 25, 2007 from ttp://www.standardprocess.com/history.asp

Eck, P., Wilson, L., (1988). *Nutritional aspect of stress.* Retrieved March 1, 2008 from http;//www.wrltma.com/stressdoc.htm

Eck, P., Wilson, L., (1991). *Nutritional aspects of depression.* Retrieved March 1, 2008 from http//www.arltma.com/depressiondoc.htm

Eck, P., Wilson, L., (1993). Fatigue. *analytical research labs, inc.* Retrieved March 1, 2008 from http://www.arltma.com/fatigue doc.html

Eck, P., Wilson, L., (1997). Adrenal burnout syndrome: *analytical research lab,* Retrieved June 14, 2006 from http://www.arltma. com/burnoutdoc.htm

Eck, P., Wilson, L., (1997). *Adrenal insufficiency.* Retrieved June 14, 2006 from http://www.arltma/AdrenalInsufDoc.htm

Encyclopedia, Britannica. (2008). Acetate: pathways in steroid hormone biosynthesis: online art. Encyclopedia Britannica Online. Retrieved February 28, 2008 from http:www.britannica.com

Enersen, O. D., (1994). *Hans Hugo Bruno Selye.* Retrieved February 24, 2008 from http://www.whonamedit.com/doctor.cfm/2538.html

Entringer, S., Kumsta, R., Hellhammer, DH., Wadhwa, PD., Wust, S. (2009). Prenatal exposure to maternal psychosocial stress and hpa axis regulation in young adults. *Hormones and Behavior, Feb; 55(2):292-8.Epub 2008 Nov 25.* Abstract retrieved June 13, 2009 from Pub Med data base

Epel, E., (2004). Accelerated telomere shortening in response to life stress. *Proc National Academy Science* USA, Dec 7; 101, 17312-17315. Retrieved March 9/2004, http://www.general-medicine.jwatch.org/cgi/content/full/2004/1224/4

Food Navigator.com/Europe (2000-2008). *Fast food consumption increases obesity risk.* Retrieved March 16, 2008 from http://www.foodnavigator.com/news/printNewsBis.asp?id=52305

Farr, G., (2001). *All about standard process/dr. royal lee—the legacy.* Retrieved February 26, 2008 from http://www.becomehealthynow. com/article/auppssp/166/-70k

Food and Agriculture organization of the United Nations (2003). *Increasing fruit and vegetable consumption becomes a global priority.* Retrieved March 16, 2008 from http://www.fao.org/english/news room/focu/2003/fruitveg1.htm

Foundation, G. M., (2001-2007). *The world's healthiest foods.* Retrieved October 8, 2007 from http://whfoods.com/foodstoc.php

Frost, Sullivan, (2003). *Fast food consumption and dietary intake profiles-fast food.* Retrieved March 16, 2008 from http://findarticles. com/p/articles/mi_11_111023412/print

Gaff, B., Hugel, H., Rich. P, (2001) The effects of eleutherococcus senticosus and panax ginseng on steroidal hormone indices of stress and lymphocyte subset numbers in endurance athletes. *PubMed.* Retrieved April 1, 2008 from PubMed data base

Gallagher, C., (2005). Dinning out: making better choices. *Institute for physical & sports therap.* Retrieved July 13, 2008 from http:// www.spineuniverse.com/displayarticle.php/article1132.html

Gates, D., (2006) Nourish your adrenals towards the foundation of youth. *A Grain of Salt, Summer, 2006*

Gorman, G., (2004). Fight, flight, or phantom fatigue. Nutrition Health Review: *The Consumer Medical Journal,* 2-4 Retrieved October 8, 2007 from http://web.ebscohost.com/ehost/delivery?vid= 9&hid=116&sid=62c06ac0-7da- 4d62-9cb

Goudsmit, E., (1998). Treating chronic fatigue with exercise. *British Medical Journal,* 317(7158), 599a-.

Guo, L., (2007). Effects of rehmannia glutinosa oligosaccharides on proliferation of hepg2 and insulin resistance *Zhongguo Zhong Yao Za*

Zhi, Jul (32 (13)), 1328- 1332. Abstract retrieved April 2, 2008 from http://www.biowizard.com/pmabstract.php?pmid=17879738

Gupta, N., Jones, J., Pocinki, A., Sharp, L., (2008). Respect for chronic fatigue long overdue. *The Clinical Advisor,* 2, 53-59.

Hair tissue mineral analysis. (1999). Newsletters and healthy news, Retrieved January 16, 2007 from http: www.arltma.com/hairana lysis.html

Hampton, T., (2006). Researchers find genetic clues to chronic fatigue syndrome. *Journal of the American Medical Association*

Hart, A., (1995). *Adrenaline and stress.* USA: W Publishing Group. *Healthy eating: tips for a healthy diet.* Retrieved July 13, 2008 from http://www.helpguide.org/lifehealthy_eating_diet.htm

Hellhammer, DH., Wust, S., Kudielka, BM., (2009). Salivary cortisol as a biomarker in stress research. *Psychoneuoedocrinology,* February, 34 (2): 163-71, Abstract retrieved June 13, 2009 from PubMed data base

Herbs with tonic, adaptogenic, adrenal tonic and nervine activity (*2005) MediHerb News Letter* No. 58 October

Hidden toxic metals. (1999). Newsletters and healthy news, Retrieved January 16, 2007 from http:www,arltma.com/hiddentoxicmetals news.html

Hillen, T., Schaub, A., Hiestermann, et.all., (1999). Self-rating of health is associated with stressful life events, social support and residency in east and west berlin shortly after the fall of the wall. *Journal Epidermal Community Health* 2000, August 575-580. Retrieved March 8, 2008 http://www.jech.bmj.com/cgi/content/abstract/54/8/575?maxtoshow=&HITS=10&hits=10&RES

Holmes, M., (2006). Adrenal fatigue——the effects of stress and high cortisol levels. Retrieved May 24, 2006 from http/www.womento women.com/adreanalfatigue/index.asp

Hutjens, M. (2005). U.S. Dairy Consumption. *University of Illinois,* Retrieved April 12, 2009 from http://www.livestocktrail.uiuc.edu/ dairynet/paperdisplay.cfm?contentID=7447

Hywood, A. N. (2004). *Stress management paper* presented at the Standard Process Lyceum 2004, Lake Geneva, Wis.

Ilyia, E., (1989) Adrenal stress index. *Diagnos-Techs, p.1-43*

Institute of Heartmath, (2001). *Emotional balance and health.* Retrieved September 16, 2007 from http://www.heartmath.org/printer- friendly/print-research-soh-27.html

Isaacs, S. M. F., FACE (2002). *Hormonal balance.* Boulder: Bull Publishing Company.

Jeffcoate, W., (1999). Chronic fatigue syndrome and functional hypoa- drenia-fighting vainly the old ennul. *The Lancet* 353 (9151). 424- 425. Retrieved March 9, 2008, from http://www.thelanet. com/journals/lancet/article/PIIS0149673698003250/fulltext

Kincaid, Joseph, (2004). *Application of Clinical Nutrition in the Practice,* Standard Process Lyceum 2004, 56-72

Kitchen, J., (2001). *Townsend letter for doctors and patients.* October, 2001 Retrieved March 25, 2008

Komaroff, A., (2001). Mild hypocortisolism confirmed in chronic fatigue syndrome. *Journal Watch.* Abstract retrieved March 9, 2008 from http://general-medicine.jwatch.org/cgi/content/full2001/ 427/2

Kiecolt-Glaser, J., (2003). Chronic stress and age-related increases in the proinflammatory cytokine IL-6. *Proc National Academy Science,*

9090- 9095. Retrieved March 9, 2008 from http://general-medi-cine.jwatch.org/cgi/content/full/2003/805/4

Lam, M., (2002). *Adrenal fatigue.*1-37. Retrieved June 13, 2006, from http://www.drlam.com/A3R_brief_in_doc_format/adrenal_fatigue .cfm.

Lang, J., (2004). *Functional endocrinology part III.* Paper presented at the Functional Endocrinology.

Lang, J., (2002-2007). *Balancing male steroid hormones naturally* Paper presented at the Functional Endocrinology

Lang, J., (2007). *What to do about sweet and carb cravings.* Paper presented at the Balancing Male Steroid Hormones Naturally, Moline, Il 61265.

Lawrie, S. M., & Pelosi, A. J., (1996). Essential elements of the treatment must be identified. *British Medical Journal,* 312(7038), 1097a-.

Leese, G., (1996). Short-term night-shift working mimics the pituitary-adrenocortical dysfunction in chronic fatigue syndrome. *Journal of Clinical Endocrinology & Metabolism* 81, 1867-1870. Retrieved March 15, 2008 from http://jcem.endojournals.org/cgi/content/ abstract/81/5/1867

Leshin, M., (1982). Acute adrenal insufficiency: recognition, management, and prevention. *Urology Clinical North America.* 9(2), 229-35 Abstract retrieved January 25, 2007 from PubMed data base

Leventhal, H. P.-M., Linda; Leventhal, Elain A., (1998). It's long-term stressors that take a toll. *Health Psychology,* Vol. 17 (3), 211-213.

Liberti, L., (1978). Inside the stressed out. *Journal Pharmacy Science,* 67 (10), 1487- 1489. LTd., T. A. C. (2004). [Electronic Version]. Retrieved June 6, 2008

Life Extension (1995-2008). *Adrenal disease.* Retrieved March 2, 2008 from http://www.lef.org/LEFCMS/aspx/printversionMagic.aspx? CmsID=39582

Lovas, K., Huseby, ES., (2007). Salivary cortisol in adrenal disease. *Tidsskr Nor Laegeforen,* March 15; 127 (6): 730-2 Abstract retrieved June 13, 2009 from PubMed data base

Lovera, I., Roit, Z., Duggal, S. (2006) Sudden death of a young woman after months of fatigue. *The Clinical Advisor 99, 98-99*

Lucile Parkard Children's Hospital (2006). *Diabetes & other endocrine and metabolic disorders.* Retrieved June 4, 2006 from http//www./pch.org/diseasehealth-info/healthlibary/diabetesdaaghub.html

Luong, D., Watts, C., Koon, A., Kooper, J. (2007). Primary adrenal insufficiency. *Consultant Live,* 11, 1180-1181

Low adrenal function/adrenal insufficiency (2006). Retrieved June 13, 2006 from http://www.diagnose-me.com/cond/C17669.html

Mayo clinic healthy weight pyramid: a sample menu (2008) Retrieved July 13, 2008 from http://www.revolutionhealth.com/healthy-living/food-nutritio/healthy-weight-pyramid?id

Mc Craty, R., (2003). *The scientific role of the heart in learning and performance.* Institute of HeartMath, 1-10

McKenzie, R., O'Fallon, A., Dale, J., Demitrack, M., Sharma, G., Deloria, M., et al. (1998). Low-dose hydrocortisone for treatment of chronic fatigue syndrome: a randomized controlled trial. *Journal of the American Medical Association.*

Herbs with tonic, adaptogenic, adrenal tonic and nervine activity *(2005) MediHerb News Letter* No. 58 October

Melamed, S., Shirom, A., Toker, S., Berliner, S., & Shapira, I., (2006). Burnout and risk of cardiovascular disease: evidence, possible causal paths, and promising research directions. *Psychological Bulletin*, 132(3), 327.

Mercola, J., (2001). Overactive *adrenals leads to insomnia*: Mercola.com. Retrieved November 7, 2005 from http://www.mercola.com/2001/aug/29/insomnia.htm

Mercola, J., (2000). *Understanding adrenal function*. Retrieved June 6, 2005 from http://www.mercola.com/feigi/pf/2000/aug/27/adrenals.htm

National Center for Complementary and Alternative Medicine (2006). *Disease or condition*. Retrieved March, 24, 2006 from http:/www./nccam.nih.gov/health/bydisease.htm.

National Center for Complementary and Alternative Medicine Medicine, (2006). *What is complementary and alternative medicine?* Retrieved May 24, 2008 from http://www.nccam.nih.gov/health/whatiscam/

National Center for Complementary and Alternative Medicine (2005). *Dr. hans selye performs seminal stress research*. Retrieved February 24, 2008 from http://www.thenewmedicine.org/timeline/stress_research.

National Institute of Health (2006). *Niacin (vitamin b3)*. Retrieved April 15, 2008 from http://www.nlm.nih.gov/medlineplus/druginfo/natural/patient-niacin.html

National Institute of Health (2006). *Pantothenic acid (vitamin b5)*. Retrieved April 15, 2008 from http://www.nlm.gov/medlineplus/druginfo/natural/patient-vitaminb5.html

National Institute of Health (2006). *Vitamin b6*. Retrieved April 10, 2008 from http://www.nlm.gov/medlineplus/druginfo/natural/patient-b6.html

National Institute of Health Medline Plus. (2006). *Licorice (glycyrrhiza glabra l.) and (deglycrrhizinated licorice)* Retrieved October 18, 2007 from http://www.nlm.gov/medlineplus/druginfo/natural/patient-patient-licorice.html

Natelson, B. H. (2001). Chronic fatigue syndrome. *Journal of the American Medical Association,* 285(20), 2557-2559.

National Center and Alternative for Complementary and Alternative Medicine (2002). *What is complementary and alternative medicine.* Retrieved May 24, 2006 from http://www.nccam.nih.gov/health/whatiscam/

National Center and Alternative for Complementary and Alternative Medicine (2005). *Magnesium,* Retrieved October 7, 2007 from http://www.ods.od.nih.gov/factsheets/magnesium

National Institute of Health (2005). *Medical encyclopedia adrenal glands.* Retrieved June 4, 2006 from http://www.nlm.nih.gov/medlineplus/ency/images/8720.htm.

National Institute of Health. (2004). Medical encyclopedia: *Addison's disease.* Retrieved June 6, 2006 from http://www.nlm.nih.gov/medlineplus/print/ency/article/000378.htm

National Institute of Health. (2005). Medical Encyclopedia: hypoglycemia. *U.S. National Library of Medicine and National Institutes of Health.* Retrieved June 42006 from http://www.nlm.nih.gov/medlineplus/print/ency/article/000386.htm

National Institutes of Health, (2006). *Dietary supplement fact sheet: vitamin B12,* Retrieved October 7, 2007 from http://ods.od.nih.gov/factsheets/vitaminb12.asp

Nerozzi, D., (1989). Early cortisol escape phenomena reversed by phosphatidyl serine in elderly normal subjects. *Clinical Trails Journals,* 26.

Newall, A., Anderson, L., Phillipson, J.D., (1997). *Herbal Medicines.* London: The Pharmaceutical

News Target (2004-2005). *Systems of medicine explained: conventional, alternative, complementary and more.* Retrieved May 26, 2006 from http://www.newstarget.com/019365.html

Nippolt, T,. (2009) *Adrenal fatigue:what causes it?* Retrieved January 23, 2011 from http://www.mayoclinic.com/health/adrenal-fatigue/ AN01583

Normal Endocrine Surgery Clinic (1997-2002). *Diseases of the adrenal cortex.* Retrieved June 4, 2006 from http://www.endocrineweb.com/ obesity.html

Normal Endocrine Surgery Clinic (1997-2002). *X-ray test for adrenal gland tumors.* Retrieved June 6, 2006 from Http://www.endro crineweb.com/adrtest.html

Normal Endocrine Surgery Clinic (2002). *Diseases of adrenal cortex cushing syndrome* [Electronic Version]. Retrieved June 4, 2006.

Normal Endocrine Surgery Clinic (2002). Your adrenal glands [Electronic Version]. Retrieved June 4, 2006

Ostatnikova, D., (2002). Salivary testosterone levels in preadolescent children. *British Medical Journal Pediatrics,* 1471-2431. Retrieved March 20, 2008 from http:www.biomedcentral.com/1471-2431/2/5

Pawlak, L., (2007). *Emotion, stress, and disease.* Paper presented at the Institute for Natural Resources, Des Moines, Iowa

Pawlak, L., (2007), *Stop gaining weigh.* Concord: BioMed General

Payaytty, S., (2007). Human adrenal glands secrete vitamin c in response to adrenocortictrophic hormone. *American Journal Clinical Nutrition.* 86(1), 145-149.

Peta, B., Complementary aid, *Times, the United Kingdom.*

Pfadt, E., & Carlson, D. S. (2006)., Acute adrenal crisis. *Nursing,* 36(8), 80-80.

Pick, M., (1989-2006). *Women's alternative health care——how to make it work for you. Women to women.* Retrieved May 5, 2006 from http://www.womantowoman.com/womenshealth/integrativehealth care.asp?id=1&campai gnno=alternative

Pick, M., (1998-2008). *DHEA and adrenal fatigue.* Retrieved March 2, 2008 from http://www.womentowomen.com/adrealfatigue/dhea.aspx? id=1&campaignn0

Powell, P., Bentall, R. P., Nye, F. J., & Edwards, R. H. T. (2001). Randomized controlled trial of patient education to encourage graded exercise in chronic fatigue syndrome. *British Medical Journal,* 322(7283), 387-.

Prevention, C. f. a. (2006). *CFS possible causes.* Retrieved 10/1, 2007 from http://www.cdc.gov/print.do?url=http:www.cdc.gov/cfs/cfs cauuses.htm

Prins, J., Meer, J., Bleijenberg, G., (2006). Chronic fatigue syndrome. *The Lancet,* 367 (9507) 346-355, Retrieved March 9, 2008 from http://www.thelancet.com/journals/lancet/article/PIIS0140673606 680732/fulltext

Reid, S., Chalder, T., Cleare, A., Hotopf, M., & Wessely, S. (2000). Extracts from "clinical evidence": chronic fatigue syndrome. *British Medical Journal,* 320(7230), 292-296.

Robbins, J., (2004) *Application of Clinical Nutrition in the Practice,* Standard Process Lyceum 2004, 20-32

Rosen, B., (2007). *NutritionIndex* . [Electronic Version]. Retrieved July 15, 2008

Salvatori, R., (2005). Adrenal insufficiency. *Journal of the American Medical Association*, 294(19), 2481-2488. Retieved October 14,2007 from ttp://jama.ama-assn.org/cgilcontent/abstract/294/19/2481?maxtoshow=+HITS=10+hits

Selye, H., Earle, R. (2008). *Canadian institute of stress.*

Shames, R., Shames, K., (2005). *Feeling fat, fuzzy, or frazzled.* United States of America: Hudson Street Press

Shannon, J. B. (2002). *Stress-related disorders sourcebook* (First Ed.). Detroit: Omnigraphics.

Shepherd, C., Macintyre, A., Franklin, A. J., Sadler, M., Goudsmit, E. M., White, P. D., et al. (1997). Graded exercise in chronic fatigue syndrome. *British Medical Journal*, 315, 947

Shifren, J. L., (2004). The Role of androgens in female sexual dysfunction. *Mayo Clinic Proceedings*, 79(4), S19-S24.

Shirotsuki K., Izawa, S., Sugaya N., Yamada KC., Ogawa Y.,et al. (2009). Salivary cortisol and dhea reactivity to psychosocial stress in socially anxious males. *Internal Journal of Psychophysiology*, May: 72(2):198-203. Epub 2008 Dec 24, Abstact retrieved June 13, 2009 from PubMed data base

St. Germain, R., Yigit, S., Wells, L., Giratto, J., Salazar, J., (2007). Cushing syndrome and severe adrenal suppression caused by fluticasone and protease inhibitor combination in an HIV-infected adolescent. *AIDS Patient Care & STDs*, 21, 373-377.

Straus, S. E., (1996). Chronic fatigue syndrome. *British Medical Journal*, 313(7061), 831-832.

Streeten, D. H. P. (1998). The nature of chronic fatigue. *Journal of the American Medical Association*, 280(12), 1094-1095.

Stress, C. I. O., (2000). *Biographical information for hans selye, CC, M.D., Ph.D, D.* Sc.

Sullivan, F., (2003). *Fast food consumption and dietary intake profiles-fast food.* Retrieved March 16, 2008 from http://www.findarticles.com/p/articles/mi_m0887/is_11_22_111023412

Swaab, DF., Bao AM., Lucassen PJ.,(2005) The stress system in the human brain in depression and neurodegenation. *Netherlands Institute for Brain Research.* Abstract retrieved January 25, 2007 from http://www.ncbi.nlm.nih.gov/entrez/query.fegi?itool=abstractplus &db=pubmed&cmd=retrieve&opt=ab

Talbott, S., (2002). *The cortisol connection.* Berkeley: Publishers Group West.

Tattersall, R. B., (1999). Hypoadrenia or "a bit of addison's disease." *Medical History* Oct 43, 450-467. Retrieved March 15, 2008 from http://www.pubmedcentral.nih.gov/pagerender.fcgi?artid=1044180 &page&pagein dex=6.

Teitelbaum, J., (2007). From Fatigued to Fantastic. New York: Penquin Group.University of Maryland Medical Center *Endocrinology health guide the adrenal glands* [Electronic Version]. Retrieved June 4, 2006.

Tindle, H., Davis, R., Phillips, R., Eisenberg, D.,(1997-2002) Trends in use of complementary and alternative medicine by US Adults. *Alternative Therapies.* Jan/Feb, 2005 Vol.11, No.1 p.42-49

Truth about environmental illness. (2004) *British Medical Journal,* 317(7163), 957a-.University of Maryland Medical Center *Endocrinology health guide underactive adrenal glands/ addison's disease.* Retrieved June 4, 2006.from http:www.UOMM.edu/endocrine/cushing.htm

Understanding adrenal function (2000). *Diagnos-Techs* [Electronic Version], Retrieved June 6, 2005.

University of Maryland Medical Center (2004). *Endrocrinology health guide adrenal tumors* [Electronic Version]. Retrieved June 4, 2006.

University of Maryland Medical Center (2004). *Endrocrinology health guide overactive adrenal glands/ cushing's syndrome* [Electronic Version]. Retrieved June 4, 2006.

University of Maryland Medical Center (2004). *Endocrine health guide underactive adrenal glands/addison's disease.* Retrieved June 4, 2006 from http://www.umm.edu/endocrine//addison.htmUS National Library of Medicine,

United States National Institute of Health (2006). *Cushing's syndrome.* Retrieved June 4, 2006 from http://www.nlm.nih.gov/medline plus/print/ency/article/000410.htm.

Wallace, M. T., Svahn, D. S., Loudon, M., & Skloot, F., (1998). Seeking answers to chronic fatigue syndrome. *Journal of the American Medical Association,* 279(21), 1697-1698.

Waves, A., (2001). Trends in U.S. per capita consumption of dairy products, 1909 to 2001. *US Department of agriculture economic research service.* Retrieved April 12, 2009 from http://www.ersusda.gov/AmberWaves/Scrips/prints.asp?page=/June03/DataFeature/

Weil, A., (2005). Ask Dr. Weil. *Prevention,* 57(12), 74-75.

Wetzel, M., Eisenberg, D, Kaptchuk, O., (1998, September 2). Courses involving complementary and alternative medicine at us medical schools. Journal of the American Medical Association, Vol 280, 784-787.

Wilson, J., (2001). *Adrenal fatigue the 21st century stress syndrome* (First ed.). Petaluma: Smart Publications

Wilson, J., (2002). *About adrenal fatigue: adrenal fatigue.org.* Retrieved June 14, 2006 from http://www.adrenalfatigue.org/whatis.php

Wilson, L., (2005) *Adrenal burnout syndrome.* Retrieved September 25, 2006 from http://educate-yourself.org/cn/adrenalburnout19apr05.shtml

Wilson, L., (2008). *Brain fog.* Retrieved March 2, 2008 from http://www.drlwilson.com/articles/brain_fog.htm

Wilson, L., *The hair analysis interpretation handbook.* Phoenix: Analytical Research Labs, Inc.

Wolbeek, M., et all. (2008) Glucocorticoid sensitivity of immune cells in severely fatigued adolescent girls: a longitudinal study. *Science direct.* Abstract. Retrieved March 10, 2008 from http://www.sciencedirect.com/science?_ob=ArticleURL&_udi=B6TBX-4RR216F-1&_use

Woods, J., (1957). The effects of long-term exposure to cold upon adrenal weight and ascorbic acid content in wild and domesticated norway rats. *The Journal of Physiolgy* 135 (2), 384-389.

World Health Organization, (2005). *Promoting fruit and vegetable consumption around the world.* Retrieved April 11, 2009 from http:www.who.int/dietphysicalactivity/fruit/en/print.html

Wu, Z., Luo, J., Zeqi, L., Luguang, (2005). American ginseng modulates pancreatic beta cell activities. *Chinese Medicine* 2007, 2:11.

Yaneva, M., (2004). Midnight salivary cortisol for initial diagnosis of Cushing's syndrome of various causes. *Journal of Clinical Endocrinology & Metabolism,* 3345-3351. Retrieved March 20, 2008, from jcem.endojournals.org

CPSIA information can be obtained at www.ICGtesting.com
Printed in the USA
LVOW110025090512

280935LV00005B/2/P